FOR LOVE OF ANNE

The poignant story of a mother's struggle to save her dying daughter

Translated by Robert Bullen and Rosette Letellier

FOR LOVE OF ANNE

by Claude de Leusse

David McKay Company, Inc., New York

First published in France, 1972, as *Le dernier jour de Juillet*
First American edition, 1973
Designed by Paula Wiener
ISBN: 0-679-50423-0

LIBRARY OF CONGRESS CATALOG CARD NUMBER: 73-84067
MANUFACTURED IN THE UNITED STATES OF AMERICA

to Zoulette

Foreword

There are books that are entirely a kind of happy expression. Ask about the author, she was not a writer. She was simply a human being who one day felt a compulsion to speak. This need, felt in each of us to varying degrees, finds here its perfect tone and sticks to it. Dangers inherent in such ambition—lack of tempo, self-pity, melodrama—are surmounted without guile and without concession, in an aura of ingenuousness and easy grace that fills us with admiration. Here is a stark book, divested of sentimentality, true to the point of cruelty—one must always face up to the cruel and the dumb—offered to our emotions like a beautiful *ex-voto* with charming colors and in its sorrow a noble pride. A slice of life, and tears clouded by sweet laughter.

Without fear of lessening Claude de Leusse's achievement, I must add that there is nothing to wonder at: a happy expression is always dictated to us—here dictated by Anne, and we read this book as we would an amorous dialogue pursued beyond death, a vibrant thanksgiving to the frail creature who in her very weakness, because of her weakness, knew how to teach her mother all about living.

Those who knew Anne, so beautiful and so modest, wounded from her earliest years, facing a dead-end life with a quiet courage few adults would be capable of, will recognize her voice. Those who did not know her will sense her, extraordinarily alive. They'll see revived a grave and reserved little girl who never ceases being a child, playing, waiting for her mother's homecomings, a girl who accepts with a melancholy reserve not being part of the life of her older sisters. They will also discover —because mother and daughter are of the same flesh— how fragile is despair and how strong is hope against all reason.

When we come away from a book like this, it stays with us forever; everything seems rather pale to us; but a profound certainty remains: love for our children is a magic balm, it transforms our sorrows, colors our joys. It alone gives us the right to raise our heads a little. Its lovely light is the privilege of those few hearts who accept with equal force the inevitable and the illusion.

Michel Déon

FOR LOVE OF ANNE

I

ANNE WAS BEAUTIFUL, courageous, and so very unassuming.

She was love and tenderness. She was a sweet child and smart.

She had a funny, rough voice. A slight build. A pure and romantic face. She also had an exquisite, out-of-date, timeless courtesy. After all, as Jouhandeau says, saintliness may be nothing but the height of politeness.

We loved each other madly.

Death came, like a monstrous deceit, interrupting everything. The everything that had hardly begun.

It happened the last day in July, quietly, in a deserted Paris.

Anne was barely fifteen.

This last day—July 31, 1970—began at three in the morning. We hadn't been apart that whole month of July. I wanted so to make up for those absences of mine, they saddened you so. Every morning, you came into my room and asked in your deep voice, "Will you come home for lunch? Will you be home for dinner?," and if I said yes, you'd say, "Fine." Your little face would light up and you'd add, "That's nice."

And if I said no, you'd also say, "Fine," but add, "That's too bad." It broke my heart, but we went no further.

Many times lately I had had to postpone getting home from a trip, and—to avoid hearing your distant voice saying on the phone, "That's too bad," or else, "You're too much"—coward that I was, I sent a telegram.

We always tried to comfort each other.

You hid your pains and nausea from me. Also your sadness sometimes at not being able to do what others did, to live the same life as your two sisters or any little girl your age.

And I did my best never to be sad, never to show you the anxiety that churned within me.

Every time the doctor left the house, or we left the hospital after a consultation, you watched for the expression in my eyes. I used to say—and besides it was sometimes true—"He's very pleased; he says everything is all right."

Then we would kiss each other madly, and laugh and make plans.

From the time the disease began, more than thirteen years ago, we took on the habit, come what may, of living between "remission" and relapse, between hope and doubt. Yet we never came to know despair.

We cheated a little. We cheated often. That was the game. The essential condition of our game of happiness. But we weren't fools. Only accomplices.

For nearly six weeks, Anne had been practically unable to eat or drink a thing. The few mouthfuls of water she quietly sipped with a straw or the few spoonfuls of yogurt she tried hard to swallow came right back up almost at once. Then she would slip into the bathroom and turn the lock so nobody could see her vomit. So she wouldn't upset anyone. When I was not home, Anne asked Zoulette, her beloved confidante, to tell me when I got back that she had eaten a very good lunch or dinner. And I pretended to believe it.

That night then, when I came home, I found Anne in my big bed.

You often made yourself at home in my bed. My room was larger, more cheerful and convenient than yours. But you always returned to sleep in your own little bed.

That night, you stayed. You were sleeping lightly. Your breathing was short. I watched the vein in your frail neck beat precipitately. I watched you. That pure profile of yours moved me more than ever: your little face, sharpened by sickness, with those immense, deep-set, clear eyes that were sometimes the color of water, sometimes of the sky.

Thank God, there were no more traces of those fat, artificial cheeks that years of cortisone had given you—that monstrous drug that had swollen your slight body out of all proportion and torn your skin.

You had suffered so from putting on that excess weight. It didn't belong with you, and sometimes people ridiculed you sarcastically.

Oh, how I wanted things to be different! How I wanted to protect you from it all.

Anne was soon to suffer from her adolescent concern with her appearance. Sometimes she didn't even want to look at herself in the mirror. "How long will it take for me to be thin again?" "Soon, soon . . ." It was no longer easy keeping her in clothes, covering up those fake curves, the terrible havoc wrought by Cortancyl—something however that she could not live without.

I looked at your hands . . . those long, long, narrow hands with their fingers so thin that we likened them to spaghetti.

I stretched out beside you and took your tiny wrist into my hand. Your pulse was going wild.

When he put the stethoscope on your heart, a few days ago, the doctor said something about a "gallop rhythm."

I kept looking at you, and my heart swelled with joy to see how beautiful you were, to find you again as you were before.

When you opened your eyes, I said, "How beautiful you are." You smiled and then pursed your lips as if to say, "What difference does it make?" I wondered why. Had you the feeling something was about to happen? Had you lost that marvelous faith that had never forsaken us? Were you feeling so tired now that you refused to fight? No, I don't think so.

Yet you didn't even ask me to scratch your back, the way you did every night before you fell off to sleep.

You took the little basin you'd been keeping by your side day after day, night after night. I held your forehead as you made terrible efforts to empty your poor stomach, already completely empty. Then you fell back onto your little pillow with the blue flowers. Beads of sweat stood out on your forehead and matted your hair. Daylight was beginning to filter through the shutters.

I knew that none of the many physicians, pediatricians, specialists who had attended Anne from the start of her mysterious illness were around.

Paris had emptied. It was July 31. Friday. The start of a weekend. Vacation time. In France, the month of August is dead time. Everything closes. Or almost everything: factories, stores, restaurants, theaters. Recent attempts at staggering vacations have not succeeded, and everyone leaves the city at once. It is not without a certain charm. But . . .

From the beginning of the month we had made a burrow of our house, and we were happy.

You read a lot. You loved Chinese, Russian, and Persian tales. I think our favorite book was *The Treasure of the Nibelungs.* The character of strong Brünnhilde, who had strung up King Gunther of the Burgundians on their wedding night and had him hung to a nail on the outside wall of the palace so she could get a good sleep, delighted us. "She must have been pretty damn strong," you said and then added, "I'll never do that to my husband."

We listened to music. You loved the Bach *Aria* in jazz by the "Ekseption."

I put my ear gently on your heart. Why was it beating so wildly now? It had always held out so bravely. Why that "gallop" sound? I buried my face in your long, soft neck. Here too I heard your heart pounding. How I wished we could go to sleep this way, curled up, breathing in your scent, your warmth. But your heart pounding and pounding made so much noise! It scared me.

So at seven in the morning I decided to call Dr. L's replacement. Dr. L was a nice man; he always came to the house but, oh, God, he too had left on vacation the day before.

His replacement's answering service said he wasn't

available until eight but that "in case of emergency" I should call Dr. So-and-So.

I didn't call the replacement's replacement because I knew he was not familiar with the case.

At eight o'clock sharp I called the replacement again. He was still on answering service. I redialed the number every five minutes. At nine thirty the doctor was still not answering his own number.

For all the charming little smiles Anne tried to direct my way as I leaned over her, I had the feeling she was growing weaker.

So I called the hospital. I asked for Professor X's ward. The Professor had gone on vacation and also all his assistants who had attended and known Anne for the past several years. A very gracious nurse told me she'd try to find "the doctors" and call me back.

Which she did a few moments later.

She asked me then to bring Anne in, since none of the doctors was allowed to leave the hospital.

I explained that Anne was very weak and that even an ambulance ride would exhaust her, physically, of course, but even more, psychologically.

"Hospitalization" had become an obsession with Anne. Every time she'd been told "it's for two or three days" it lasted several weeks.

How I hated to deceive her, she who had such confidence in me! She who always thought I was able to solve everything. . . .

I was really in a quandary. Should I call an ambulance? But what would I tell Anne so as not to upset her? Should I wait a little longer? Wait for what? So often we had dreaded the worst and so often her incredible vitality had got the better of the disease and of our despair. Why not this time as well?

One thought haunted me. I kept remembering how, a little more than two years before, Professor Z, who had taken care of Anne from the first symptoms of her illness, had asked me to come in alone.

Very gently he made me understand that from then on Anne could not be expected to live more than eighteen months or two years. . . . Therefore it was no use putting her to the pain of all the treatments, those innumerable drugs that were destroying her digestive system, her bones, her blood. Anne was then on a very strict diet, and this kind and humane man added, "Let her eat what she likes, take her on a trip, make her happy."

And for a week I was terribly tortured, torn between going away with her, to have our fling, to do everything that had always been forbidden, the sun, the sea, boating, long motorbike rides. . . . To let her stuff herself with crude foods, pretzels and junk, to put salt and sorrel on everything, to drink all she wanted . . . even to go out to discothèques, like Castel's or Régine's, to go to bed no matter how late . . . to do everything and laugh and love each other and never be apart for a single moment.

And then the fear of being wrong, of precipitating an end that was not inevitable. It settled over me. Had I the right to relinquish the fight we had been carrying on for eleven years? We knew we had to play for time, because new remedies were constantly being found, because one day they'd find the one that would cure this disease. Then too I was confident; I believed in life; I did not believe in surrender, in giving up. I did not believe in fatality; I didn't know despair. And finally, finally she was just a child, how could a child die?

So I sought the advice of another specialist. He had the reputation for being a "fighter" . . . and things went on.

That's what I was thinking of, and of what Anne had answered yesterday when, seeing her thoughtful, big eyes gazing into space, I asked, "What are you thinking of?" "I'm thinking of everything I could have done if I hadn't been sick," she answered. It hurt me so to have refused her the trip back to Spetsai that we had been planning on, and to have canceled the three-day boat ride I had promised her.

She took everything with such infinite grace. We had decided to go to our good old Corrèze as soon as she felt better. We'd go to Chamboulive everyday on motorbikes and go mushrooming, for chanterelles, with Tonton, her tiny dachshund, himself the color of a rich brown mushroom. "And you'll stay with me all summer?" Yes, I promised to stay with her all summer and not to go to work. Then, all smiles, Anne added, "You're so right"; she took her pillow under her arm and went off to watch television.

That was yesterday . . . July 30.

The ring of the telephone interrupts my thoughts. It's the hospital nurse announcing that a doctor will finally come. I tell Anne. He has an Oriental name.

"I know him," she says.

Of course she does, she knows so many of them.

At about ten-thirty he arrives. He's pleasant; he has a deep, soft voice. He leads me into the drawing room. All I hear from his monologue are two words that ring in my head as a verdict of capital punishment must to a convict . . . "terminal stage."

However, to be certain that we are going into the

"terminal stage," the child will have to be transported to the Hôpital des Enfants Malades for involved tests, which I know too well, and "to perfuse her."

I suggest that this time the intravenous feedings be done at home. The doctor shakes his head; it's impossible.

So I ask him to explain it all to Anne.

He goes into my bedroom, sits on the edge of the big bed, takes her frail little hand into his broad hands, pats hers gently, and, with much kindliness and in great detail, explains to Anne that it's important that she go to the hospital in order to regain her strength.

Anne listens. She curls up the corners of her mouth, meaning, "Okay, if that's the way things are . . ."

The doctor promises she'll be back home Monday.

At the door, he adds kindly, "I'll keep in touch with the interns and stop by to see her Monday morning."

It's a fact. It is Friday today and doctors don't go to the hospital on weekends.

I return to the bedroom. Anne heaves a sigh and wrinkles the tip of her nose.

I say, "When you get out of the hospital, we'll go to La Chèze. You know they'll make you feel better, don't you? Remember the time you couldn't speak, you got your voice back when you were there. Now you can't eat; well, there you will."

"You'll bring me home on Monday?"

"Cross my heart."

One morning three years before, Anne woke up unable to speak. Zoulette ran for me in a panic. Anne was trying to say something and could emit only inarticulate sounds. She was making a terrible effort but not one intelligible word came out of her mouth. Her eyes filled with terror, incomprehension. I'll never forget the anguished, questioning look on her face.

I handed her a piece of paper and a pencil.

"Write what you want to say."

She tried with great care, but she was unable to form any letters and the pencil slipped out of her fingers.

Anne then threw herself down on her pillow and big tears rolled down her cheeks.

I hugged her to me and covered her with kisses.

"Be calm. It'll pass. Don't worry, love . . ."

An ambulance came right away to take her to the Hôpital des Enfants Malades.

As soon as you arrived, Anne, do you remember? a group of doctors and nurses surrounded you, seemingly very calm. But they were concerned. They asked you questions and quickly taught you how to answer yes or no. You opened your hand to say yes, you closed it to say no. And it became a game.

Eight hours later, suddenly, you turned to the nurse and said very clearly, "I'm thirsty."

"Say that again," said the nurse, releasing the bottle she held in her hand.

"I said, I'm thirsty," you repeated, triumphant.

We kissed each other, all of us.

All traces of paralysis had disappeared, never to return.

They talked about a small blood vessel bursting in the brain, of hypertension. . . . They didn't really know.

We order an ambulance. It's eleven o'clock.

At eleven-thirty, two strapping men in white smocks come to get Anne. They have an air of "Oh, boy, everything's great!" that gets on my nerves. One of them grabs Anne under the arms. She seems to be in pain. I know how sore she is, but she doesn't say a word.

She's wearing the blue nightgown with puffed sleeves and a little bow at the throat. The bow keeps coming undone. It's hot.

During the ride, she motions to me discreetly that she is becoming nauseated. But she holds back and doesn't flinch till Rue de Sèvres. I hold her very slim, hot hand in mine; the pulse is very fast.

My sister-in-law, Kakoze, is in the front seat, squeezed between the two attendants.

Once again we go through the big stone hospital gate. On the pediment, engraved in big gold letters, "Hôpital des Enfans *[sic]* Malades." Below, in red letters, "Liberté Égalité Fraternité."

I often wondered why the word "enfans" had no "t." I never remembered to ask. I'll probably never know. What difference does it make?

They send us to Chaumont ward. We know Netter, Aviragnet, and many other pavilions. Chaumont is a small white pavilion, to the left as you go up the central hall. It occurs to me we won't have to walk so far when we come to see Anne.

It is noon.

The little canteen wagons, pulled by an electric cart, meander through the pavilions, tintinnabulating.

It's lunchtime.

They settle Anne on the second floor, in one of those cubicles, glassed in on three sides. There's a window with no way to open it, a radiator, a small washstand, a chair, a metal night table.

Not all the nearby beds are occupied. In summer the hospital is never full.

The children who can walk draw near to have a look. The boldest of them press their noses to the door.

"Hi, what's your name?" says a dark-haired little girl. Anne smiles back but doesn't have the strength to answer.

A black nurse comes into the ward nonchalantly pushing a cart loaded with plates of mashed potatoes, bowls of stewed fruit and dishes bouncing around.

The children go back to their places and spoons rattle against plates.

Anne is stretched out, motionless, her eyes opened wide and turned toward the window. I can see that she's very weary, that all she wants in the world is to be left alone. How I regret suddenly having brought her here! Now we are caught up in the infernal rigamarole of blood samples, X-rays, transfusions, perfusions. And the examinations, the taking of her temperature and blood pressure, with no let-up. The suffering, the physical pain. I want so much to protect her from all that.

They remove her chain, her medal, and the little Brazilian good luck *figa* that she is never without; also her big plastic watch that I place right near her on the table so she'll be able to see the time.

She always wants to know what time it is. She has an extremely keen interest in time. In her room there are several calendars and every night, before going to bed, she goes from one to the other crossing off the day that has passed.

A nurse comes in, hands a thermometer to Anne, takes her blood pressure, writes something on the metal-framed chart and leaves without a word.

Now I have to go fill out the ritual entry forms. I hurry down the stairs and run up to the entrance. A young man mumbles the usual questions: "Has the father been told? . . . Who will come to pick her up? . . . Do you have the means to pay forty-five francs a day? . . ." and, "Sign here under 'authorization to operate.' "

I sign.

Then I rush to the Health Services office. They waste no time. They know her file.

When I return, several blood samples have already been taken from Anne. She seems resigned; she knows they're going to bother her, but she also knows it's for her own good. For the moment, all this activity reassures her.

A tall, skinny intern whom I haven't seen before enters the cubicle to examine Anne. Then he asks me to follow him into the office at the entrance to the ward. He looks shy and he's obviously not familiar with the case. Must I once again tell all about the disease and its thirteen years of ups and downs? It occurs to me that we haven't much time now and that something has to be done quickly. I answer his questions as precisely and quickly as I can. He seems extremely puzzled and anxious. Of course, I understand, I know: it's not a simple case.

We go back to Anne. He looks at her a long time. Then a small, dark-haired woman with a round and gentle face comes in. She examines Anne too. After a while, she runs the tips of her fingers lightly over the big eyelids and the deep circles under her eyes and whispers:

"She's quite sunken . . ."

This awful word strikes me smack in the face. The woman intern looks at me. I look aside. I want to hide the damned tears. Softly, she repeats, "She's quite sunken."

Someone comes for another blood sample. Glass tubes are filled and more blood is needed for the slides.

They make an incision at the tiny tip of each of her fingers, and squeeze and squeeze some more to collect the little red drops. They're all white, her "spaghetti."

Anne's little face is twisted in pain, but she doesn't say a word.

I feel like strangling the intern.

No one bats an eye.

When the intern leaves, Anne tells me:

"I feel sick."

"Nauseated?"

She shakes her head "no."

"Your head? Your tummy? Are you thirsty?"

She slowly shakes her head at each of my questions; she parts her lips but says nothing. Her breathing is more and more jerky.

Nanou, I love you.

I so wish I could do something to make you feel better. I abhor it, this impotence. What's the good of love then? What's the good of life?

I could give you my blood and keep just enough for myself, just enough to continue the fight and my life with you, close to you. I want you to live. I'll give you everything I've got. I'll never leave you again for a single instant.

A short Negro comes in. He's there to do a chest X-ray. At first Anne refuses to sit up. I think she's in pain and wants to be left alone. We help her to sit up. She looks so tired.

And what if I take her away in my arms, away from

here, so they can't torment her anymore? Dear God! Why did we come? Why did I call this morning? Why all these torments? Why?

Results arrive by the minute now . . . very low calcemia . . . high urea count . . . liver very enlarged . . . infiltrated lungs. . . .

It's four o'clock.

A huge nurse, the fat of her legs wrinkling and folding over her ankles, comes heavily into the cubicle, dragging her feet. She looks a good sort.

She carries the bottle for the intravenous medicines.

She bumps into everything, shakes the bed, drops things.

She takes Anne's frail little arm into her huge hand and says:

"You have pretty veins."

I look at the bluish streaks running under the transparent skin.

The giant takes a needle and pricks her, pricks again, turns the needle, rummaging around in the flesh.

Anne throws me a resigned, painful look.

At last the needle is in, and the fat woman realizes that it is plugged up.

She tries to pump with the tube and the needle comes out. I feel a homicidal madness rising in me.

Then the nurse decides to try the forearm. And here it goes again. She searches for the little vein that slips, withdraws. She perspires. Anne too. Me too.

It goes on forever.

At last she pricks the back of the thin little hand.

There it goes. Blood all over the place.

Then, when she plugs into the bottle, the drip doesn't

come. Fatso gets nervous, her feet get tangled up in the night table.

The tall intern pokes his head through the door and says:

"Fourteen drops a minute."

I watch the drops fall one after the other. I expect that Anne will regain her strength very soon.

But after a few minutes her heart begins suddenly to beat faster. Very fast. Too fast.

The artery in the neck throbs and the little bow on her nightgown leaps in the same rhythm. Her breathing grows more and more rapid.

I'm scared.

The intern slows the tempo of the drip. Kakoze is back. Her presence is a comfort. She's always there when you need her. Anne and I love her.

I sit on the radiator. Instinctively I look before I sit down. . . .

Once, during one of the numerous stays at this hospital, Anne was in a very large ward of forty beds, in the big building at the end of the central mall.

She had been doing cutouts; I put them in a paper bag and placed it on the radiator. The next day, when I turned the bag over for her to go back to her cutouts, a swarm of cockroaches fell on the bed. Anne wasn't upset and laughed when she said:

"I'm used to it."

She saw my disgusted look and added:

"It doesn't matter. Don't say anything."

As usual I didn't, but I went to the nurse and asked for an insect spray. She looked sheepish and answered:

"We're allowed only one aerosol can a week per ward."

The next day I brought a carton of aerosol bombs and all our able-bodied little friends in the ward went hunting cockroaches.

It was during the same stay that I found Anne one morning with the upper part of her arm swollen, bulging enormously. During the night the needle for the perfusion had slipped and all the liquid had flowed into the tissue of the arm. Anne was too little to realize. And anyway she never complained.

I went to tell the intern on duty about it. His answer made me shudder:

"We only have one head nurse at night. It's a shame. There's nothing we can do about it. She can't do the job."

I offered to stay the night.

"That's not allowed," was the answer.

One head nurse for forty sick children . . . and the battle waged by the doctors of the urology ward to get an extra kidney machine. . . .

There was also that other summer—it was always during the summer that severe relapses occurred—when I had left on a trip. When I got back, I found Anne completely immured in a cast on her hospital bed. Only her skinny little arms and her long toes poked out of her ghastly mold. The cast had been so hurriedly made that it hurt Anne everywhere. She was chafed under both arms and on her feet. When I asked the reason for all this, the intern on duty, who had ordered it done, answered that they were afraid of osteomyelitis. It's true, Anne had had dubious pains in the tibia of her right leg. So, in order to immobilize that one leg, they had shut her up in a cast almost totally.

What's more, Anne had her right arm immobilized by a perfusion. She was left-handed. Charles, her father, had asked that the cast be cut to loosen it on the chest and under the arms. When I arrived I pleaded with them to open it on both sides.

A few days later I brought Anne home.

When I took her out of her shell to give her some relief, she was so reasonable that she wouldn't move a bit, but her face lit up with gratitude.

Anne really never recovered from that long immobility. From that time on, she never walked with ease again. She lost a toenail that never quite grew back.

Doubt engendered revolt in me. Of course, I didn't let it show. You just don't want to think that suffering like that is useless.

Anne coughs.

Her short breathing turns to a whistle.

Her big blue eyes are uneasy.

Suddenly she takes a breath and says:

"Don't forget to water my plant," and then:

"You'll wind my alarm clock."

Her last words.

The short, dark-haired intern is back. She seems worried. "We're going to give her oxygen, it'll help," she says.

The giant nurse doesn't know how the oxygen valve works.

"I've been here thirty years," she says. "But this isn't my department. I'm a substitute here because of all the construction going on. I know how to set up the oxygen tent but this gadget isn't my thing."

All groans and grumbles, she finally gets "the gadget to work."

Consincienciously, Anne holds the little funnel in her good hand and presses it to her mouth.

"Does it help?"

She nods "yes."

It's after six. The tall, dark-haired intern comes to get me. He talks about dialysis and purifying. I know what that means. The kidneys are working less and less well. The blood will have to be purified with the "washing machine." Softly he says:

"It's a little painful . . . a big needle in the peritoneum. . . . We can't put her to sleep, her heart is too weak."

The idea that Anne will suffer again horrifies me.

"You're sure we have to?"

He's nice; he twists a piece of his smock in his hands. I feel dizzy.

"I'm not completely sure," he says. "The intern in charge will be here in a moment. We'll see. In any case we'll put her there for the night."

What if I made a violent objection?

But a glow of hope flickers in my heart.

Everything is confused.

I say nothing. I return to my little girl. I dampen her lips with a compress.

The "intern in charge" has come. I'm called into his office. He's a short, red-haired man with a self-satisfied air.

"Why have you brought her so late?" he says dryly.

I don't answer.

The tall, dark-haired intern is back with me in the cubicle. Very gently he explains to Anne what will be done.

She frowns and looks at me. I say something to comfort her. I tell her I won't leave the hospital that night, that she'll feel better the following morning. She breathes the oxygen through her little funnel.

As usual, she accepts. She is calm. She is beautiful.

At about eight that evening, a short attendant comes to fetch her. He puts her on a cart. The perfusion bottle swings from the jolting and I keep my eye on the needle. I'm afraid it'll come out. But it doesn't budge on the white hand that is tied to a small board. Anne still holds the oxygen funnel tightly.

We go up the central mall, we turn to the left and then to the right. It is getting dark. There's not a soul about, all is silent.

We enter the long pavilion where Aviragnet ward is and also the consulting room we've been coming to almost every month, Wednesday mornings, with Zoulette.

We cross ominous, very dark hallways. Then the little black nurse, who never stops smiling, pushes the cart into a big elevator. Kakoze and I cling to the rear wall. We go up to the second floor.

It's the artificial kidney ward.

We go into a room where the heat is overwhelming. There are two beds.

A little boy about four years old is asleep in one of them. He is tied down and pipes come out from everywhere. Near him, a big machine, a kind of electronic console, purrs. Anne looks at the child.

Also in the room is a tall, skinny nurse. She throws a

sour look our way and doesn't say a word. On her face, there's none of the smiling kindness common to nurses. I hope Anne hasn't noticed.

The nurse settles Anne in the other bed, near the window. She pays no attention to her. Not a word, not a smile. I try to balance Anne's watch on a tiny table near the bed so she'll be able to see the time.

"There's no room for that kind of thing here," says the nurse, removing the watch.

Timidly I ask her if she would please slip the little white-and-blue cushion we brought with us under Anne's head.

"She doesn't need it," she answers brutally.

Anne looks at me and smiles. Meaning, "I don't need it; it doesn't matter, don't say anything."

I say nothing.

I go into the hallway for a moment. I run into the short, red-haired intern. I ask:

"Are you going to operate?"

"Of course," he answers and disappears into another room.

Kindly, the tall intern tells me:

"It'll take about half an hour; you can come back then."

The little, dark-haired one is there too. She smiles at me.

I go inside to see Anne. The tall bitch of a nurse has planted herself in front of the bed. I want to beg her to give me just a moment to kiss Anne, to take her in my arms. I'd like to tell her that she's in pain, that she's docile and courageous . . . that she's very ill . . . that . . . maybe she'll die tonight.

Of course I don't say a word.

Nothing gets through this dark and hostile face. The look of her eyes, her attitude, her every movement is a reproach for my presence.

She didn't let me get close to the bed.

She looked at her watch.

I think she was annoyed that so difficult a case was brought to her at nine at night.

I tried to find excuses for her, and probably she had enough of them: she was tired, it was late . . . maybe her shift was over and she'd been asked to work overtime? Maybe she had a date? Maybe she was going on vacation?

But why such hostility? It was beyond me.

Anne—Mme Zouk, my Nanou—Grand Duchess of Gerolstein (as your father used to call you), I wanted at that moment to give you every drop of sweetness and tenderness in the world.

So at the door I said:

"See you in a little while. I'll be right out here. I'll be back soon."

Love words were what I wanted to say.

You watched me leave. A long, very sweet look. You smiled. You put on your "don't worry, everything will be fine" look. You wanted to comfort me. How good you are. How brave. How I love you.

And I left.

Kakoze took my hand and we walked the empty paths. We didn't speak. We went through the hospital gate and into a small café just about to close. I asked for two telephone tokens and a Coca-Cola. I called home. The big children, Caroline and Laurence, were supposed to leave for Spetsai the next morning. I told them they'd have to wait. I didn't know what to say. Kakoze wanted me to eat a sandwich. We shredded little bits of ham that we weren't able to swallow.

And we returned to the ward. It was dark. The air was warm.

The door to the room is closed.

There's nobody in the corridor. I'd like to see someone, to get some news.

Suddenly, the nice tall intern comes out of the room and closes the door right away. There are many people inside.

Kindly he says, "Don't stay here please. It's going to take a while longer."

Kakoze gets me to go to a friend's house nearby. She gives the intern the phone number; he promises to call as soon as the operation is over.

I remember taking off our shoes and nibbling fresh almonds at the friend's.

I called up Charles. He wanted details, explanations. I don't think he fully realized. I told him to come to the hospital a little later. I know he hates it. I'd like to spare him that.

How can I manage to spare them again?

And Zoulette? She left two days ago for her little house in Binic. I'll call her tomorrow morning. She'll return at once. Anne will be pleased.

They'll play *crapette.*

Also, I'll build another mobile and we'll hang it on the ceiling of your bedroom.

When we got back to the hospital, the tall intern said: "It's over. But Anne is very hot, because of the sterile fields. You must wait a little while before you see her." And he vanished.

I sat on a step at the foot of the stairs. Through the

windowpane I saw the construction site, some planks, a tree. I smoked. One cigarette after another. I was thinking of nothing. I wondered why I was thinking of nothing.

My brother, Guy, came then. He sat down very close to me on the step. How did he guess? I don't know; I didn't ask him. We always knew everything about each other without having to say much. It was good to feel him there. We smoked and smoked. I ground out the butts under my sandals.

The waiting smothered us.

Toward ten, I went up to the little office. Anne's belongings were in a corner. The office was closer to the room she was in. I wanted so for someone to tell me something. I wanted so to see her.

Then I heard a long-drawn-out whimper. I still hear it. I will always hear it.

The little, dark-haired intern came up, wrapped in a pinkish brown apron. She seemed sad. She says, "The child is doing very poorly. . . . We're going to put her into resuscitation."

There's no resuscitation equipment in the building we're in.

White smocks run about in the night. Run to find the resuscitation apparatus. Wherever it is. Somewhere else. In another building.

The equipment is rolled in. At last. With a big noise. The doors close again. That's all. Silence.

I go back to sit on the steps. In the half shadow. In sadness.

I hope now it's all over.

I don't want her to suffer anymore.

I say to Guy:

"I want to take her to Chamboulive."

"Of course."

I think that there's only one vacant place in the little cemetery, that it was one of our summer jokes around the big table at La Chèze; that my grandmother and grandfather used to argue good-humoredly about it; that my mother, practical and to the point, would put an end to our lame jokes by saying that there were plenty of available places in the big family vault at Tulle.

However . . . however I'm sure I don't really believe that Anne is going to die.

The little intern has come back to say that heart massage is being done.

Then toward midnight she says: "We did everything we could."

I ask if I can see Anne.

I'm told that I still have to wait.

Then the black nurse came by. She said that we could go and sit in a waiting room on the second floor—belated, derisive attention. She was wearing a light dress. She walked fast. She was going home. She was off duty.

Anne is dead.

It is midnight.

I went to put a kiss on her lips.

No more looks from those blue eyes. No more sense of shame. Nothing but tears. And infinite emptiness.

They'll put her in that dreadful little gray building out back. The morgue.

I went home.

I watered your plant.

I wound your alarm clock.

II

AND THEN THERE WERE all those things that kept us apart. That kept me from you. And they are the ways of man.

All those material things that seem to be made to drive into your head and heart the repellent reality of death. Something like a wide and final break.

It took me months to wind up again the tenuous thread of thoughts and memories that link me to you. That thread is my indelible treasure. It's your presence coming from elsewhere.

The next day. The first morning, when I emerged from a short, drugged sleep with the mad hope that it wasn't true.

The first morning without you. Without your voice . . . your warmth . . . your presence.

The void. The vertigo. A terrible lack. A violent, carnal pain. The total disinterest toward everything else. The love for life that has gone with life and love.

But also that dreadful revolt that snarls inside you when confronted with an injustice that nothing can explain. So renunciation was my lot. But I didn't accept. I'll never be able to.

And those questions that never stop coming back, haunting and painful. Those thoughts that seized my insides. Why didn't they let her go quietly? Why didn't they let her die tenderly? Why that final brutality? Why wasn't I there, beside her, next to her, with her? Why did I agree? Why?

Two reasons, however, like two props, forced me not to give in. First, the two other children, "the two big ones." Then she, who never wanted to hurt anyone and whom my sadness would have distressed.

One time, just once, I had let myself go and I cried in front of you. I had hidden my face in your neck, beneath your hair, but you noticed anyway. You hugged me so tight that time, almost strangling me, and you said in your deep, throaty voice, "Poor Mother." And you added, "Don't be upset. Life is not so sad."

Yes, that's what *you* said. And I said: "Poor Zouzou, your mother is completely off her rocker."

We burst out laughing and talked nonsense. But I saw that your eyes were full of tears.

I felt ashamed. I told myself "never again."

This morning. Saturday. August 1.

Kakoze has come to pick me up early. Guy has joined us. I want to do everything myself. I need precise jobs to do. I want to do everything as it should be done.

Nanou, you hated disorder, imprecision, delays. You dreaded the unforeseen, fantasy, the unexpected. At home, we didn't exactly lead what can be called a regular life. It was rather a peculiar life that hardly fitted into the norms of what a bourgeois family takes for granted. You were often surprised, upset. But your forbearance, sick little girl that you were, was amazing. Especially toward me. You always took my side. Your problems you entrusted to Zoulette. My job was to solve them.

I sent a cryptic message to Zoulette in Binic. She understood right away. She's taking the train and will arrive this afternoon.

She had only you. She loved only you. She defended you fiercely and paid attention only to members of the family who showed you any tenderness and who gave you a little of their time. Poor dear Zoulette. On August 15 she'll be seventy-three years old, and you won't be here to help her blow out her birthday candles.

I chose a nightgown. The one with a large, round collar and high cuffs, the one that made you look like a (blond) Velázquez infanta.

I took it to the hospital, to the Administration Building. A man said to me, "I'm sorry," and he had me sign the death certificate. He told me to take it to the funeral services office in the municipal building of the Fifteenth Arrondissement. He gave me, rolled into a ball, the little blue nightgown Anne was wearing yesterday.

I went to the municipal building. The doors were open. I asked for the funeral services office and was told it was closed until Monday and that in all probability, and because of the reduced staff during the month of August, nothing could be done before Tuesday.

There was a stone in my stomach.

No doubt about it, one should not die on the eve of a weekend, and never on the first weekend in August.

Then we looked everywhere, all over the hospital, for the chaplain. Nowhere to be found. My brother and Kakoze spent hours running from one church to another, from one parish to another, trying to find a priest. In vain. There didn't seem to be a priest available in Paris, that Saturday, the first of August, to come and bless Anne. Anne so pure, so pious. I knew she didn't need it anyway. All the same. It was hard to believe.

Therefore we decided to call the Borniol people. A composed gentleman came to the house. He asked many questions, punctuating each with an apology. It was a matter of wood, lead, white satin, cross. Price. I had always wondered how these things could be "settled." And today, here I was on the drawing room sofa, the place where Anne always watched television, making decisions about her burial and its details. I felt outside myself and at the same time terribly clearheaded. I kept wondering, looking at this stranger in mourning clothes, how a person could choose a job like that and be led as he was to make a living on death. There was no animosity in the thought, merely curiosity. I think I even felt a kind of admiration for this man who must harvest only absurd hatred and saddened indifference in his job.

Everything was settled for Tuesday, August 4.

Late in the afternoon, I returned to the hospital. I wanted to see Anne. Kakoze went with me. We took the back road, a little dirt path running alongside the old Necker Hospital. In front of the dreadful little gray building I stood perplexed. Would I have the courage to knock at those handleless wooden doors, with a rusted key in the lock? Did I really want to go in? The ground was dirty. Nearby a shed gave cover to a hodgepodge of tools. No one ever seemed to come this way. It was the abandoned section people avoid. I was scared.

At last a man in a smock came by. He hesitated and said, "Whom do you want to see?"

"Anne de Leusse."

"A few minutes, please. You can sit on the bench."

He went inside through one of the wooden doors and closed it behind him. We sat down on a peeling old bench between the two doors. We didn't say a word.

My first thought was that a morgue couldn't look more ramshackle in the heart of what they call an "underdeveloped country." I thought "morgue" a peculiarly ugly and pretentious word. I thought of *Black Orpheus.* I thought too that till now the word only evoked detective stories in my mind.

The man in the smock reappeared. He said, "Who are you?" I said, "Her mother." He gave me a smile and nodded for me to go in.

I hesitated. My heart was pounding. Fast. Strong.

We entered a dark, cold little room. Anne lay on a high, narrow bed, to the right along the wall. Behind the bed was another door. I imagined the depth of cold, of darkness, silence, solitude. I shivered.

Mme Zouk, Anne, my love, my baby, how beautiful you were.

Anne wore her infanta nightgown. Her little wooden cross and her little gold *figa* hung at the end of her chain.

A hand, I guessed whose, had already put a little bouquet of pink roses between your long fingers.

I put her little magazine *Nade* down beside her and a letter that had just arrived by mail that morning.

I kissed her icy forehead; there were beads of water on it.

You were like a flower, Anne, in the morning dew.

The man said, "Don't touch her. You understand, in all this heat. . . ." All right, he's doing his job.

I leave. I flee.

I wish someone would hit me over the head to keep me from thinking. Keep me from imagining. How far will the pain go?

What are the limits of the unbearable?

I wanted nothing anymore. Nothing.

Not music. Nor the lovely light. Nor beautiful words.

I thought of something Léon Bloy had written: "*In the face of a child's death, art and poetry come to resemble a great destitution.*"

Life had become totally empty.

I didn't go back there. Until very early Tuesday morning.

The chaplain was there. He said prayers.

I placed a love letter beside Anne.

They closed the coffin.

They placed her in a black hearse. It was covered with white and pink roses.

And we took the long way. Not the one we used to take. One that was more to the east.

For hundreds of miles I never took my eyes off the black car. From time to time we lost sight of it because it was going too fast. I'd feel an anguish in my heart then. The heat was suffocating. In some places the road shone as if there were puddles of water. The murky air danced. Charles, drove. He had loosened the knot of his black tie. Zoulette, Caroline, and Laurence were in the rear. We spoke very little. We made attempts to say nice, trivial things to one another. To make it easier. To forget for an instant.

We were very hot in our black clothing.

The immense fields of freshly cut wheat of Beauce looked like doormats. The corn was high and the big suns of the rape nodded. Not a breath was there to shake them.

Around one in the afternoon we reached the roads of Creuse, cool, winding, big trees on either side. We were always losing sight of the black car because of the curves.

At Treignac I sat next to the driver of the hearse to show him the way. We crossed the Chamboulive square, swarming with people. They were waiting for us. It was past three. We didn't stop.

I wanted to go one more time to La Chèze with you. Two miles of road, every bend, every hedge, path, almost every stone of which was familiar and concealed childhood memories: the grade crossing that we sometimes forgot to close; Gourdon Lane to the left with its big black firs; Bel-Aspect Road on the right from which a herd of cows often emerged; and then the short stretch going straight down where we used to ride our bikes at top speed; Mal Val Lane at the entrance to which there once was a sign saying *Mas-le-Val* which didn't, however, drive away the evil morning fogs that lurked at the bottom of the little valley; and Levesne Bridge that crosses Rujoux Brook where we used to fish for crayfish, gudgeons, and shiners—the last my father's favorite, fried—and even trout under the stumps. After Levesne Bridge there is a big climb that the huskiest of us could make to the top on our bikes, standing up; on the "green knoll," to the right, on a curve, there is an old barn unused forever that is said to be haunted. We cycled around that curve racing to the point of breathlessness because we were so scared. Finally the narrow road that climbs to La Chèze. My grandmother, Mamy, would say, "A quarter of a mile to go." "It's a good half-mile," my father would retort and we would settle for a third. That's what the sign says.

We passed by the Benissou. Old Mme Bessoul was at her window between her pots of geraniums.

And then the pond. And then the bakehouse covered with reeds. We circled the "cake" of flowers. We stopped a while beneath the locust. The white shutters of the house were closed. My grandmother was seated on a bench, in front of the library. She had stayed there alone. She was crying. She came toward us in small steps, leaning on her cane. She kissed the coffin.

Tonton, Anne's little dog, jumped into the car. He was happy to see me. I pressed him to my heart. He gave my salted cheeks a big lick of the tongue.

Then we went back down.

The old church was cool. Flowers everywhere. There were all the familiar faces of this countryside I love. All the women from the village and from the farms round about.

Guy, Eric, Jean-Pierre, André carried the coffin. Aunt Zizi played the Bach *Aria* you loved (she didn't know that it was your favorite) on the harmonium. We were very moved.

I remember that the priest, in his colorful burr of an accent, said very simple and beautiful things. I don't remember what, though.

Climbing to the cemetery, Yvette and Solange, the twins from the farm, Sophie and three other little girls, your friends, were the pallbearers, the pall was white. They sobbed. I remember that passing in front of the Deshors Café there were two vacationers, naked to the waist, drinking. They watched the long column pass by and went on chatting. For a moment I thought they were totally out of keeping and indecent.

But I didn't give a damn. After all.

Marc was so sad Uncle Guy took him to Leyris's to buy him a new bicycle with racing handlebars.

And there were the hundreds of letters. Letters of affection, love, tenderness, friendship. Only one of them spoke of "deliverance" and I didn't answer it. It was too absurd.

And those long months of agitation when I scattered myself deliberately. Work. Trips. Long nights without sleep, seeking some shelter. Obstinately destroying myself. Vodka in Russia. *Cachaca* in Brazil. Scotch anywhere. Getting drunk. Morning bitterness. Dreadful awakenings, my face bloated and burned by tears. I looked at the "accordion pleats" around my eyes ("You remember our jokes, Zouk?"). Every morning a song went around in my head, "When you cry you grow old, that's life, don't let it get you down, lalala, lalala."

Don't let it get you down. How?

I never liked mornings in a house. The windows open, the drafts, the noise of the vacuum cleaner.

Now I hated them. I got out fast.

I did things one after the other. I was concerned by everything and nothing. I fled solitude and silence.

Everything served to lead to oblivion.

However, Anne, I had gusts of you that hurt. When I came upon one of your familiar objects, an image, a sound, everything inside me came to a stop.

At first I even wanted to give up the apartment. I was unable to go into your room. I was afraid to open your drawers, your white wardrobe and the chest filled with your games and all that make up the treasure of a little girl. I was afraid to see all the mobiles dance from your ceiling—the straw birds, the little silver fish, the watches, the green dragon, the clouds, the sailboats, the parasols of many colors, each of these things representing a stay in the hospital and careful work. The mobiles came to life in the drafts and I can remember you watching them dreamily while you lay down resting on your bed.

Finally, of course, I decided to stay.

Suddenly it seemed cowardly to surrender your little kingdom to alien and indifferent hands, unbearable to destroy it or to try to erase it. It soon became clear that I could never leave a place that spoke of you. On the contrary, little by little, I set about seeking such places. They made me feel good.

I let memories rise up again. I no longer defended myself against them. I no longer tried to protect myself. I let you enter my life again.

And I found you again.

III

ANNE WAS BORN quietly at the end of a hot weekend in early summer.

The name we really gave her was Anne-Christine, but we called her that very rarely if at all. Only when we wanted to be a little pompous.

She wasn't expected so soon. She wasn't really expected.

She was so slight it was almost as if she wanted to apologize for being another girl, or simply for having come.

Her hair and her eyes were as light as her sisters' were dark. She had long, very narrow feet that punctuated shapely little legs at right angles. Some people compared her to a comma, others to a fork, still others to a romantic miniature.

She was so fine and delicate her father called her "the grand duchess."

We didn't mind her being another girl. We had decided it was more fun to form a collection. My sister-in-law told Caroline, because she wasn't permitted to come up, that there was no staircase at the clinic, and I introduced her little sister to her through the window.

Caroline was three years old. Laurence was just eleven months. Caroline was both gentle and authoritarian; Laurence, spontaneous and violent, and she had a thirst for knowledge that was very tiring though it made us laugh. With the coming of Anne, her big problem—let's say of identification—was born. For years we came to say, based on her being either with Caroline or with Anne, "the two big ones" or "the two little ones." Her strong personality had good reason to suffer from this and very soon she learned to say, "I can't thtand that" when we called to her as part of one pair or the other, or she simply didn't answer, since neither pair really applied to her.

Anne like her sisters was baptized at Senlis Cathedral. Her godfather and godmother spent an afternoon at Valgenceuse under the shady trees in a large park, eating Jordan almonds and simpering over the cradle. Anne stared at them with her immense blue eyes but she didn't give them one smile; maybe she knew they weren't good fairies. At any rate, we never saw them again. There was also a distinguished old uncle who mistook me for the nanny. I was delighted and took advantage of it by taking off.

Then we piled up baby bottles, diapers, suitcases, straw hats, sandpails, and shovels and thousands of other things in the Citroën and we went off to spend the summer at my parents' house, La Chèze, in Central France. Caroline counted Shell stations and tirelessly sang, "I lost my little kerchief as I strolled down Indian Street." Laurence said *no* to everything, she refused to sit or lie down and fell asleep standing up squeezed between knees and bundles.

Orléans, Vierzon, Châteauroux, Limoges, Uzerche,

how many times! The curves tossing the children one over the other, the screaming, the quarreling; a slap that ends in the air—"mith'd!" Laurence would lisp in triumph. Our patience wore out with the miles.

We arrived at last and the hubbub would be at its peak. What we needed was never in the suitcase we opened. Children were all over, my brother's children, the children from the farm. They dashed to the sand to make mud pies and throw them in each other's eyes. My mother had gone to "tremendous trouble" to clean up the house for our coming and instantly the disorder was indescribable.

She ran everywhere, left and right, trying to gather little shoes and tiny red boots into pairs, to mop up the water from a spilled vase, to pick up the pieces from a broken toy. Her beauty was equal to her efficiency. Equable and constant.

Though they were all about the same age, almost none of the children ate the same thing. What's more, everyone's schedule was different.

Which meant that there was always one woman or another in the kitchen washing baby clothes in warm water, diapers in boiling water, stirring cereal, or cooking a chop.

A nightmare that time has made seem funny.

Even more, at that time, we had to draw water in buckets from the well all day long.

In the evenings, we pulled a small zinc tub up before the *cantou* (the big fireplace of the region, high enough to stand in) and we plunged the children into it two by two.

The three girls slept in "the big room," the one above the dining room and just as spacious. There were at least four beds there, not including the cradles.

We had all lived there at one time or another. We called it "the gypsy's room." We knew all its nooks and crannies, the big, wooden nail-studded wardrobes, the huge gold-framed mirror hanging by a menacing string that no one ever tested. And then there were the noises: from the roof, the mice "tenants" who tirelessly moved God knows what around all night; the regular crunch-crunch of the little worms eating into the hardwood floor; and then, early every morning, the creaking of the shutters that were opened from downstairs, the door beating back and forth, and the other that nobody was ever able to shut without slamming.

Anne often cried during the night, and in order for her not to waken the others we brought her cradle down to the library when everybody had gone to bed.

One night we were hit by a storm of an unheard-of violence.

The day had been scorching hot.

All the white wooden shutters were closed. Bees were buzzing in the grapevines.

In the evening, everything stopped. We couldn't hear the bullfrogs croak. The dogs didn't bark. Not a breath of air shook the leaves. The silence was anguishingly thick.

With night came a continuous roll of thunder and flashes of lightning from all directions. We had the feeling of being in the exact center of a narrowing ring of fire. It lasted for hours. Not a drop of rain fell. Before vanishing silently, as on every night, Mamy said, "Dry storms are the worst." And we all went to bed. But in the middle of the night we were awakened by the sound of an infernal bellows. The shivering of the slates made me rush down from my garret; I thought the whole thing was going to fly away.

I ran to the library door. There was such a suction from the draft that two of us pulling with all our strength, braced against it, had a hard time opening the door.

Anne was asleep.

On the staircase was a procession of nightgowns and pajamas, each carrying a candlestick and making the blown-up shadows flicker.

I pressed my nose to one of the windows whose shutter had been torn away and was struck with amazement to see a heavy plank going by, blown along like a straw.

Everything was cracking—branches, trees.

The flashes of lightning brought heaps of leaves and flowers, all kinds of debris, into view. It was terrifying. There were such noises, rumbling, crackling, tearing, we wondered whether the old house would hold out.

In the early morning, we all gathered out front, our noses to the air. Our trees which surround, even embrace the house, had all suffered.

We knew perfectly well that their proximity was dangerous, that their leaves clogged the gutters every fall and their branches broke the slates. But it was out of the question to get rid of them. We had to fell an enormous oak a few years before, because there was only one alternative—it or the house—and it was a tragedy in the family. We still talked about it.

That morning the locust looked more like some Chinese tree. The maple—"it's a liquidambar," my father always specifies—was plucked clean. The huge cedar was intact but it seemed slightly bent by the rough battle of the night.

As for the chestnut, it was crippled from having lost its finest branch, which had fallen onto the roof of the barn. There was a large gaping hole. So my brother decided to have it felled. There was no other solution. The rest of it would have fallen onto the house in the next gust of wind.

It proved to be a finicky business. Paul Bordes climbed like a cat to tie a steel rope to the top of the tree and had it pulled with a winch carefully directing the fall. It collapsed with a tremendous noise. We spared everything that had to be avoided, the wall, the barn, the house and the well.

That evening the tree was sawed up and put away, out of sight. But not forgotten.

"I absolutely forbid anyone to touch a single tree on the estate," my father had often repeated. He wasn't there that day and no one ever convinced him of the necessity of our undertaking.

The children had found it all great fun. They clambered about everywhere, made small heaps of leaves and chestnuts, and then forgot the whole thing.

They went fishing with my father in Mal Val Brook. They hunted for worms that they drew out by sprinkling a little Clorox in likely spots. When one came out, the children, reacting half in disgust, half in delight, yanked at it as at a rubberband. The worm stretched and broke. Then they piled up the little curlicues mixed with mud in the bottoms of their pails and proudly marched along with the reeds they used as fishing poles over their shoulders.

Father brought them home at nightfall all muddy and tired.

Mother said, "Georges, you don't have the slightest notion of time."

Father said, "Get off my back, damn it." Everybody knew as a fact that nothing in the world could make him want her off his back.

In the evening at dinner—we were always no fewer

than twelve at the table—the maid made at least three rounds, presenting each of us with a platter. On it sprawled seven tiny fish which we'd ceremoniously refuse, leaving them for the next in line.

The noise was deafening. Everybody talked at once. Nobody listened to what anyone else was saying. My mother asked questions but seemed never to have time to listen to answers, preoccupied as she was with the overcooked roast or the too parsimonious way Mamy had of serving herself. From time to time, someone thundered, "Be quiet!" But a moment later the hubbub grew all the louder.

On September 15, everybody returned to Paris.

The children weren't old enough yet to go to school. Still we observed vacation time. It's a habit few people give up, even with age.

For the children, winter was spent between walks in the Jardin des Poètes, Thursdays at children's parties where hysterical English nannies frightened Caroline, and Sunday mornings with Yaya—a name Caroline gave my father and which he kept—on the Enchanted River and the toboggan slides at the Jardin d'Acclimatation.

That winter we brought in a tall German-Swiss girl to take care of the children. Her eyes were too small and her mouth too thin. In spite of that she was good-looking, and she used to disappear in a huge Cadillac, which waited outside for her, when she had the day off. She was strict and entirely lacking in tenderness.

Laurence provoked her constantly and bravely faced up to her, despite threats of a spanking, yelling all her new-learned words of abuse—softened as they were by a lisp. Her favorite bad word was "bathtard." There was also, "I'll thlap you."

Anne was a very sweet baby; maybe too sweet. She didn't smile much. She studied things and people with her big blue eyes. She often cried at night and the doctor said we could give her a tranquilizer, Gardénal, once in a while.

When she was about a year old, she began sleeping a lot. And one evening, when the "two big ones" were taking a bath with the Swiss girl, I heard Laurence let out a violent howl.

I paid it no attention. It was something of an everyday occurrence.

But Caroline, who was never a tattletale, suddenly appeared, indignant, and asked me to come and see. I followed her into the bathroom. Laurence's bottom was red, black-and-blue, and covered with finger marks.

I blew my top and demanded that the "tamer" leave and do her spanking elsewhere.

Tongues started to loosen then, and I learned from a good, old Spanish woman, who every night snored against the kitchen boiler for the sake of her asthma, that every bottle of milk had been accompanied by a tablet of Gardénal. But people always talk. And hadn't that very same woman, without realizing the consequences, let a fruit juice bottle containing Clorox slip under the bathtub? A bottle that Caroline swallowed in a gulp? We'd had to shake her, make her vomit, swallow milk. Then, in relief, my first emotion passing, we joked about how she was now well disinfected inside and how her hair would get blond and her skin white.

I didn't want to think about it anymore.

Life went on like this for some time.

Caroline, age four, made drawings everywhere and read Mr. MacGregor stories or sucked her thumb dreamily while, with great delicacy, stroking the tip of her nose.

Laurence, at two, was overwhelmingly active, shaking Anne's bed violently when Anne cried, obstinately messing up things Caroline tried to keep tidy, storming around, laughing and often disappearing into the drawing room where we'd find her asleep behind the draperies or under the table. To fall asleep she used to do her "spwuttering," meaning she made bubbles on her hand by sucking her thumb.

Anne began to cry or babble at night and to sleep during the day.

So we decided to place an ad to find someone who could help.

The next day, a charming lady with fluffy white hair presented herself. Her thin glasses hardly stayed up on her pretty nose. She was pleasingly plump, she had a soft voice, quiet and polite manners. I told her, without omitting a thing, what a household was like with three little girls who were almost babies.

While talking, the two of us stealing glances at each other, I had the melancholy thought: "She's much too good. She's not for me. Too bad."

She asked a few questions and left saying that she wanted to think it over a few days and that she'd call to give me her answer.

A few days later she called and asked in her soft voice, almost apologizing, whether "the job" was still open.

That's how the "good fairy" Zoulette came into our lives.

Her bearing, the head a little in front, slightly ahead of her solid hips, her expression, her language, very soon became totally familiar to us. "Do your teeth" meant brush them, and when a child was cutting a new tooth, it was "putting one on." Also you "took" a shampoo. She often switched the verb and the object. For instance, she'd say, "I'm Anne going to make eat," or "I'm Caroline going to make work."

She let out little cries—high-pitched ha-has—when she was surprised or when she showed interest in what we were telling her. She was extremely discreet, pious, and candid. She was afraid of nothing and made little more noise than a mouse. Except that the noise of a mouse could make her lose control of her dignity. She wielded a mean fork and that was a joy to see. She liked good wine the way she liked everything good. That's what made her so good herself.

Windy nights, storms, tempests, any sound that reminded her of the sea, delighted her.

The children liked her right away. "Mademoiselle" became "Zoulette."

The "Two big ones" teased her, of course. But there were no big scenes.

Right off, Zoulette became very fond of the youngest and most vulnerable of the trio she called "Clac" (a funny name she made up out of the first letter of each name: Caroline, Laurence and Anne-Christine).

Exquisite tamer that she was, Zoulette often had to play the role of banker, too. When there wasn't any money left in the house and I declared, "Today is a day of fast and abstinence," she would pull a bill from her wallet, carefully folded in four and take care of the marketing.

Anne began to show alarming symptoms. She ate very little and thrashed so hard she often fell out of her bed. She didn't sleep much; she cried a lot. I often took her to bed with me at night, to comfort her and to let Zoulette get some rest.

Then appeared what at first we called her dizzy spells. Anne was about eighteen months old.

It was as though she had lost her balance. Her head would go forward and she'd make a circle with her arms in front of her, like a little ballerina. Her face contorted; she seemed to be in pain. It happened at any moment, and sometimes, if we didn't grab her fast enough in our arms, she'd fall to the ground as she walked.

The doctor was intrigued, anxious.

She was given sedatives, ever stronger and stronger, more and more often. Phénergan, Gardénal, Nembuthal, Epanal. Enough to stupefy the most vigorous and highly strung adult.

One day in May 1957, while he was observing Anne, the doctor said under his breath, as though asking himself a question, "Maybe it's a 'petit mal,' a form of epilepsy."

Without a word, I took Anne with me. Her hand was so narrow I held it entirely within my own. She toddled beside me. I went to the best store to buy her the prettiest coat I could find. It was in piqué, blue-and-white striped. Anne was adorable.

Revolt and anxiety seized me. Questions without any answers. Words, names that till then existed for me only in books or on other people's lips.

I was entering a universe that should never have concerned me, that seemed totally absurd to be involved in. It was not in the order of things. In my order anyway. I always thought that certain things only happen to others, like wrinkles, when you are twenty-five.

Nevertheless, the love for life, gaiety, optimism, insouciance that I had always believed in, and that Guy called my recklessness, wasn't shaken, none of it. I tried always to push things aside, even to forget whatever bothered me. My protective system worked pretty well. The sad things of life for me were like bubbles I could see at the bottom of the water and that I kept from coming to the surface.

Anne's mysterious illness, however, had begun. Nobody suspected it yet. We groped. We searched. We weighed things. We guessed.

During the month of July we made our first visits to specialists.

They put "curlers" on Anne for the encephalograms, beams of light into her eyes for the fundus examination, needles into her veins for blood samples. But there was no progress.

Anne was still taking strong doses of sedatives, and as the weeks went by we stood by petrified and watched a regression of her faculties.

She "unlearned" how to walk and talk. Little by little she forgot everything a two-year-old child knows. She didn't know how to say "Jesus" even, and that made Zoulette very unhappy. Her eyes lost their color, there was no sharpness. She seemed indifferent, dreamier.

I sometimes had the feeling she was trying to say something; she'd come up to me, hug me around the neck as strong as her frail little arms would let her, cover me with kisses, press her tiny nose to my cheek. I'd speak to her, ask her questions, ask them again. One moment she'd look at me and smile, then turn away. There was a kind of barrier in her little brain that neither she nor I could cross. And I felt an anguish, a distress rising up within me.

Was she becoming an idiot, an "innocent," as Zoulette called it, innocently?

Sometimes she made a turn around her finger and sang. Zoulette said she was dancing.

Those bottles of syrup were loathsome to me, they spoiled her brain, the way the numberless bottles of Cortisone pills and other medicines were slyly and irremediably to destroy her bones, her blood, her digestive system. Were we already at the point where there was no other possibility? No other choice?

In the autumn of that year, they discovered that Anne had renal hematuria, a nephritic syndrome. The results of the analyses were alarming. The doctor decided to hospitalize Anne.

That was October 31. It was raining.

We took with us, in addition to Anne's white pajamas, her polka-dot cotton flannel robe, her "splippers," and a silver mug and spoon, which were very soon lost.

They put Anne in a long pavilion, to the right of the hospital entrance, in a very small room with two beds. We stayed all morning with her but, when it came time for us to leave, she reached a paroxysm of despair which both broke our hearts and warmed them too. Of course she was not indifferent! It was the first time we had ever had to part from her, the first time we had left her anywhere. We were very sad.

That first day, however, was to correspond with the first surprise in this illness. And it was a good one.

In order to undergo the thousand and one examinations, smears, X-rays, analyses, all medication was suspended. And what we had thought to be a "petit mal" and its nervous manifestations vanished entirely. Totally. Forever.

How whimsical was this sickness! It would leave one place to settle suddenly in another.

A few days later, as I was seated on the edge of Anne's bed, quietly playing with her, her eyes became wide and set. She was suffocating. I rushed to get a nurse. Anne was quickly put under an oxygen tent. "Mechanical pleurisy," they told me. The disease had flashed through her lungs. Then the spleen was hit. And always the area of preference: the kidneys.

Every stage in the development of the disease was always and to the end accompanied by a redness on the cheek bones "in the shape of a butterfly," which made people remark that Anne looked good and healthy.

Anne stayed almost two months at the Hôpital des Enfants Malades. Every day we went to see her. Zoulette brought her orange juice.

Caroline and Laurence were too young to go inside. They sent their little sister drawings, toys, and small bouquets of flowers.

Anne showed an appetite for living, knowing, understanding, more and more every day. It was as though she wanted to make up for lost time. In order to avoid the daily heartbreak of our separations, I used every trick in the arsenal of the Sioux.

When it came time to leave, I'd go and get a nurse. She'd lean over Anne and shake one or the other of her stuffed animals to distract her. Then I'd go down on all fours behind the nurse and sneak out of the room. I'd only get up out in the corridor and wait a few anxious moments. Then I'd leave in a rush.

As Christmas approached we decorated the hospital windows with decals. At the end of the corridor there was a Christmas tree that they lighted up at nightfall, with the arrival of the dinner carts.

The blood tests were bad. The doctors were anxious and were making no statements yet. Was it leukemia? But no one said so. No one had settled on a diagnosis yet.

Anne came home for Christmas. That very evening, she chewed up some pieces of a broken teapot. Which much amused her sisters and alarmed Zoulette.

Anne had become very cheerful.

She went for walks in the Jardin des Poètes.

She liked Zoulette's eyeglasses and was afraid of the pharmacist.

Anne went back to the hospital almost every month till summer. She stayed there only a few days, time for the analyses to be made and to get the results. There were a number of interested doctors looking in on the case.

Finally they found out. A complicated name. There was a report to the Faculté de Médecine. I learned that there were only fifty-two cases of the disease in the world. That it had practically never been diagnosed in a child so young. Where it came from, and why, and how was not known. It was a slowly developing disease that took the form of a mysterious auto-destruction, in which, I was told, the cells of the body—brain, liver, intestines, kidneys—were attacked, first one and then another, without apparent reason; and in which the destroyed tissue was never repaired. Apparently it was caused by an overproduction of the enzyme, collagenase, and the subsequent, slow destruction of the body's connective tissues.

They began the corticoid treatment.

Anne suddenly had become a very interesting little person. And we grasped then the precariousness of her life. We accustomed ourselves even to that. We even forgot sometimes, and that was better.

As far as possible, we decided to have Anne lead a life that wouldn't make her different from others.

Laurence pushed her around a lot, a little too much perhaps, but obviously there was no way to explain things to her. Unconsciously she felt somewhat frustrated because, of course, of the greater attention we paid to her little sister. Once in a while she even invented an imaginary pain one place or another.

Therefore the doctor who came very often to see Anne also examined Laurence minutely and with high seriousness. He prescribed innocuous little tablets for her. Everything went back to normal and Laurence was delighted.

One morning, Caroline fell on the hemp rug in the corridor and cut her chin. Another time she broke her leg and everybody came to do drawings on her cast. Each of these "incidents" put Laurence into a very bad humor. She said, "It's disgusting. Nothing ever happens to *me.*" So she did silly things, provoking everyone, defying us to the point of exasperation. I understood all this and it required a lot of patience. But sometimes this was lacking. . . .

The trio quarreled a lot and often, but they stuck together against outsiders. Any attack from outside brought them immediately back together. They made a united front. Their reserve was considerable and forbade any displays of tenderness among themselves. Despite an apparent indifference they worried about one another. More even than one would imagine.

One morning, at a time when Caroline was the only one to go to school, I took the two others to do the marketing. Anne and Laurence toddled on either side of a stroller, clutching it each by a hand. Laurence wanted to change sides every minute. She'd go behind me in a rush and give a bossy rap to Anne's fingers to make her let go. So I'd take Anne in my arms and make her go over to the other side. Anne thought this procedure rather funny. To get to our covered market we had to walk a good fifteen minutes, cross three streets and a boulevard.

Inside the market we went slowly through aisles that were chock full of housewives.

The little girls wouldn't let go of the stroller now, but they seemed constantly fascinated by something happening behind us. So they tripped over crates and bumped into shopping bags. We limped through mountains of cauliflower, artichokes, and cherries.

Now and then I stopped in front of a heap of vegetables or fruit and put a paper bag, its bottom always ripping open, onto a pile in the stroller. There was always an apple or a tomato rolling to the ground and it was Laurence's pleasure to retrieve them from among a nursery of legs.

One moment, as I was rummaging in my wallet—an extraordinarily impractical one as I recall, contrary to what it was supposed to be with all its stupid pockets and compartments—and sticking a last bunch of leeks onto the top of my pyramid, I realized Anne was nowhere around. At first, I thought she had slipped off behind the counter we were standing at.

I asked the lady to have a look. Anne wasn't there. We alerted all the neighboring merchants. No one had seen her. She was so slight and agile, she must have sneaked off. But where? I abandoned the stroller and went up the center aisle, then through the side aisles.

Nothing.

I asked here and there, "Have you seen a little blond girl?" No, nobody. I didn't want to look upset and throw Laurence into a panic; she was calling Anne everywhere. I squeezed her round little hand in mine and we paced up and down that hellish market for more than thirty minutes. Then I returned to where I had started.

I assumed Anne had to be looking for us too, and scared. She didn't talk much then. She knew her name but not her address. And if she ever tried to find her way home, she'd never be able to make it. And those streets, that boulevard to cross. The cars. My God!

"And to make things easier, there are two ways out of the market," joked the lady I had talked to first.

But I had lost all sense of humor. I didn't smile. She added:

"Take it easy, sweetheart, there's a good Lord watching over the children."

I rushed off. We left the market by the same entrance. I thought that the most sensible thing to do. Anne was nowhere.

"Mother, where is Anne?" Laurence said very upset.

"I don't know but we're going to find her."

"Where?"

After several steps, out of breath, she asked again:

"Mother, is Anne lost or has she been kidnapped?"

"Don't worry. We're going to ask a nice man to find her."

I decided to go to the police station.

People were lined up silently waiting their turns at the counter.

"I'd like to see the inspector," I said to a young man flourishing a pen over a piece of paper.

"Get in line," grumbled a woman behind us.

"What's your problem?" said the young man.

"I've lost my child," I said sheepishly.

"She's not really lost, is she, Mother?" Laurence said, tugging at my arm.

"No, no."

"Come with me," said the young man.

The inspector was in his shirtsleeves and his office reeked of smoke. I told him what had happened.

"Take it easy," he said, all good humor. "That often happens. She went back home. A four-year-old is pretty smart." And he added, "If there had been an accident in traffic, we'd have been informed."

That was reassuring.

I called home. Anne wasn't there of course.

I couldn't explain to the officer that Anne was ill and wasn't too smart yet. However I told him that she was a little on the dreamy side, and he concluded:

"Go home and don't worry. If we get any news, we'll let you know."

We went back home. Riding piggyback, Laurence cried and said over and over, "We lost Anne. What are we going to tell Zoulette? What's Caroline going to say? What's Daddy going to say?"

For more than an hour I paced the house, waiting for the phone to ring.

At last they called from the police station and said that Anne was there. I rushed over with Laurence.

Going in, what we saw made us laugh: Anne was seated at a table and around it were a dozen policemen having a snack. She was very calm, smiling, leafing backwards through a copy of *Tintin.*

I learned that a lady had found Anne sitting sadly at the door to her building—it looked like ours, by the way, and was not far from it. She had talked to her but Anne hadn't answered.

That's all we were ever to know about that escapade.

The year 1960. Of course . . .

There were, of course, the daily twenty or so pills,

wafers, tablets that we crumbled into the mashed potatoes, stewed fruit and yogurt.

There were, of course, the blood tests, analyses, and constant visits from the doctor.

They were all part of our normal life now.

Anne participated in everything with enthusiasm.

She grew prettier every day and more and more sociable.

She had her little friends, such as the two little boys she often met at the Jardin des Poètes, who gallantly helped her make mud pies.

Like any little girl, she once cut her hair with nail scissors.

She caught bad colds, like everybody else.

She spilled the button box onto my bed and the bottle of cologne in the bidet.

When she got new sandals, she refused to part with them when she took her afternoon nap. She smeared every shoe she got her hands on with white shoe polish.

Perched on her highchair, she had to be pushed to the table so she could eat her chicken, her "white lamb" as she called it, and be "unpushed" when she was finished.

Caroline played "Seven Families" with her. When Laurence was angry, Anne ran for shelter into her room and slammed the door. She waited quietly for the storm to pass.

When she was just about five years old, Anne already had a good philosophy.

She disliked quarrels, screaming, noise—all were things she did her best to avoid. She always tried to settle things.

There were moments of sadness for her, when her sisters or Zoulette or I had to go out.

She used to say, "Next time, it's my turn to go," and then she always found something, or some notion to comfort her.

When we came back, she had bursts of tenderness and said many things that touched our hearts.

When she was tired, she went and lay on a bed and sucked her thumb.

One day, lying down like this, she said:

"It's sad."

"What's sad?"

"Dogs."

"Why dogs?"

"Because they have no thumbs to suck."

In October 1960, Anne went to school for the first time, and I began modeling at Chanel's.

Both of us were escaping the house to go to work. It was "back to school" for both of us.

So one morning, Zoulette took the three girls to school. Anne had been talking about it for days. She was very proud. The whole way there, though, on the graveled path around the stadium, she said over and over, "I don't want to go. Please. Please, don't make me go." She cried and she no longer wanted to carry her brand-new bookbag. She quieted down when they got there and she entered the school proudly behind her older sisters. At the entrance to the kindergarten class, a lot of little children were crying, hanging to their mothers' apron strings. Anne was dignified and entered the room without looking back.

I went to pick them up at noon, in the yellow Vespa that looked like a mustard jar. They stood up in the back seat. The two big ones gossiped about their morning.

Anne said nothing. When we got home, I noticed that she was clutching a little package in her coat pocket.

That package—vexing witness to one of those childhood tragedies you never forget—was a pair of Petit-Bateau panties, a little damp.

Anne was pure and without any cunning; and I don't think that we would ever have found in her pocket the kind of little note that we discovered somewhat later in Laurence's uniform pocket, Laurence, the fighter, who already had such a bargaining sense, such drive and savvy. "If you're not my friend no more," said the note, "I won't give you the arithmetic answers no more."

At the end of the year Laurence won the arithmetic prize. Anne got the prize for politeness.

Getting a job at Chanel's was no small matter in my family circle.

First of all, it was still a rare thing, and wondered about, for a woman to go to work.

Then, too, being a model was low work, widely despised. Horrid things were whispered about it.

It was the time though when Mademoiselle, as Coco Chanel was called, who always liked to be provocative, declared, "In England, duchesses are models, why not in France?" Therefore, breaking convention once more, she decided to add some nonprofessionals.

It was also the time when infatuation with the Chanel style was at its peak. Such a psychological phenomenon that all the girls ended by resembling one another, with their thick bangs, the black lines around their eyes extending to their temples, their cascades of necklaces, their black-tipped beige sandals and quilted bags that swung at the end of a chain from their shoulders. And, of course, the "little two-piece suit" trimmed with braid worn over a silk blouse knotted at the neck, and the chiffon scarf. All that great uniform which was copied, imitated, repeated everywhere.

Young women who first took up the challenge of modeling had to pay the price. To begin with, remarks like "What a pity to have gone to college and end up like that . . ." or "Why not be a salesgirl instead?" or else "How will you be able to stand everybody looking at you?" and "In any case, say it's all for fun . . ."

Oh yes, that's the way it was. Really annoying that a person had the nerve or lack of shame to get involved in such a thing.

People's mentality was such that those of us who had children instructed them that in case of any underhanded or ungracious sally like, "Is it true your mother's a model?" to say right back, "That's because she's prettier than yours." This, of course, did not fail to happen and it created some incidents.

Later on, several of us even received anonymous letters at Chanel's, which among other things insulted our husbands for being too easy.

We arrived at work late in the morning. The main thing was to be there before Mademoiselle, who walked superbly down Rue Cambon between eleven-thirty and twelve-thirty, but never at the same time two days in a row.

Some of the girls had an amazing instinct and always arrived a few seconds before her, some others were eternal victims, always wrong, whom Mademoiselle would systematically call for when they weren't around, and who would then be around for months without any attention being paid them.

Mademoiselle couldn't stand a woman who wasn't perfectly made up. In fact, she liked to repeat, "Every time you go out on the street, say to yourself that you're about to meet the man of your life."

The first thing we did of course when we arrived was to shadow our eyes and put bright red on our lips. The experts helped the clumsier ones.

All of a sudden, every phone in the place started to ring. That was a signal from a watchman downstairs: "Mademoiselle is coming . . ."

Then the very nice wardrobe mistresses, Mme Georgette and Mme Andrée, flitted about in the models' dressing room, helping one of us squeeze into a long-line brassiere, bringing a glass of ice water to someone else, and we, as relaxed as could be, under the circumstances, stood at attention at the landing, wrapped in our white smocks. Mademoiselle climbed the stairs lightly, her hat straight on her head, admirably elegant.

The question uppermost in our minds: Mademoiselle's mood. When it was good, the whole establishment fell under the charm of her smile. Sometimes she pinched our cheeks, made a nice remark, and invited one of us to lunch.

But when the mood was bad—and that was rather frequent—Mademoiselle found a victim and raged. Or she went by without a word, her mouth a long pen stroke across her face. And everybody in the place treaded softly.

On such days, we took off as fast as we could.

When we had lunch with her, we listened to her endless chatter, part fascinated, part tired, curled up on her suede sofa, in front of her superb, life-size statues of does.

She'd tell us anecdotes about her life, give advice, or

rail against well-known people. By tacit consent, once down the mirrored staircase we never repeated a thing. Otherwise everyone would have been having a battle with everyone else.

Some of her favorite sayings, pronounced with all the authority of her experience, were things like "If your heart is broken, get dressed up. Make up, make yourself as beautiful as possible and go out. Be seen." Or else, "Love is all that counts. When a man loves you and you love him and he asks you to paint yourself green, paint yourself green."

She called her chauffeur "the mechanic" and every other couturier a "couture-ass."

Mademoiselle Chanel knew everything, saw everything, without ever asking questions. When you had rings under your eyes and looked terrible after a wild night, she started teasing you: "You can dance and drink every night in your life, but you'll never dance and drink as much champagne as I have."

At work her ardor was unbelievable. She stayed hours cutting, recutting, pinning armholes, and never got tired as the time for the fashion shows approached.

One day, one of the models came in wearing a Chanel suit from the last season, a suit of her own. She went up to see Mademoiselle who was all fired up with work and who didn't listen to a thing the young woman had to tell her, nor to her protests as Mademoiselle grabbed the long pair of scissors that always hung from her neck and slashed the armhole, grumbling that it still wasn't close enough to the shoulder.

When the day to present the collection to the press or the buyers arrived, she'd say to those of us who were nervous before stepping beyond the Coromandel screens, "Remember that you are beautiful, you're young, and, to top it all, you're wearing my clothes." And nastily she'd add, "Look at them out there. Old, ugly, frumpy."

To my three girls, Mademoiselle Chanel was all the more glamorous a figure for being invisible. I talked about her. They wanted to see her very much. But that was out of the question. Mademoiselle didn't like children. In fact, it was a subject not to be mentioned; she ignored it, purely and simply.

Sometimes, when there was no one to take care of Anne, I took her to Rue Cambon with me. We'd give a quick hello to the salesgirls in the boutique downstairs, hurry to the second floor, two steps at a time and into the dressing room to make ourselves scarce.

There, I settled her amid the little jars and jewelry boxes which she emptied and very carefully put back in order. Or I gave her a sheet of paper which she covered with houses, all vaguely resembling La Chèze. She drew with eyeliner. Everyone was nice and thought she was very pretty.

Anne even found a second godmother there who, once in a while, took her out to dinner and to her place to sleep. That was a real treat; Anne was delighted and so proud, she thought her new godmother was very pretty. So she'd go off with her tiny suitcase, never forgetting her medicine. Her eyes shone with pleasure and she was overwhelmed with gratitude. I was too. I was so glad to see her happy.

Toward the end of 1961 and the beginning of 1962, undercurrents of internal strife, corresponding to the violent political strife in France, often divided our unruly battalion of women.

There was hardly ever an open altercation. That Mademoiselle Chanel would not have tolerated.

She herself never aired a final opinion on things. It's true she had her perverse statements about "the arrogance of the Jews," "unwarranted foreign interference," or "mankind's stupidity," but more often she just indulged in a contemptuous "pooh" and shrugged her shoulders as a comment on an O.A.S. bombing or an instance of police repression.

But politics created a greater stir downstairs. Certain faces were triumphant while others were crestfallen. The most committed sometimes even changed from their refined suits, silk blouses, and fancy sandals into bluejeans, drab sweaters, and moccasins, and left Rue Cambon to take part in demonstrations at the Bastille.

Thus, for better or for worse, they paid off the futilities of the day with the gravities of the evening.

The foreigners, Americans and South Americans, who especially enlivened the models' dressing room, didn't give a damn for all this. Their subtly complicated lives provided sufficient preoccupation.

It was during those sad times that a little girl in Anne's class, Delphine was her name, was blinded by a bomb intended for Malraux.

The children, confused and frightened, asked a lot of questions. And we knew no good answer in the face of such absurdities.

The euphoric period began to deteriorate at Chanel's. A modeling job is essentially a short-lived one, and bearable only because it is; so the girls left one after the other for another life, or another job, or another country. Besides, Mademoiselle made no effort to keep them from leaving, she herself didn't like people and things to be permanent. She was also a little tired of the "I don't give a damn" attitude that began to prevail in the house. The eccentricities of the dressing room were no longer fun for anyone. She hired models who kept more professional hours and had more professional standards.

One day, I got the urge to leave this place from which all initiative was banished and where, if you didn't take any, you ran the risk of becoming a moron.

I had been given the pompous title of first head of the showrooms, and later press agent. But in reality I had nothing to do. I had probably none of the special gifts for diplomacy and patience the place required. I suffocated in these salons where daylight never entered and where whiffs of No. 5 floated in an often unbearable heat.

One night when I was having dinner with my brother, he led me to a mirror and made me take a good look at my pale cheeks and the bags under my eyes, all of it emphasized by the heavy makeup that was now part of my way of life. In a few harsh words he made it plain that the whole thing had gone far enough.

It was the nudge I'd been waiting for.

Early the next morning I made up with special care—for the very last time—and went to await Mademoiselle's arrival.

I think I never found her so charming.

More than once I had noticed the extraordinary instinct she had for always guessing the state of mind of the person coming to speak to her. I had seen people, livid with rage, going up the stairs leading to her private apartment, determined to get everything off their chests. After a time, short or long, they'd reappear looking utterly serene. We knew that the charm had done its work, that Mademoiselle Chanel's ineffable smile had instantly melted the anger, that a thousand things had been discussed, a thousand other matters brought up except for the one the meeting was all about.

By turns she was adored and abhorred. She jolted you with tenderness, hatred, laughter, anger, admiration. She revolted you and fascinated you. There were no lukewarm feelings where she was concerned.

When I left her that morning, she said cryptically, nicely pinching my ear, "I know what kind of a woman you are!" and, at the threshold of the heavy glass door, she added, "Come back whenever you like, if you like." She had on her marvelous smile.

I was a little confused. Both delighted and sad to be free. Strongly determined anyway not to come back, ever.

It was August 1962. In October I started with *Women's Wear Daily,* the bible of the American fashion industry. I was a fashion and features correspondent for Paris, and as fashion is more than just a hemline, is a way of life to WWD, we had to cover everything.

For two years, Anne had been attending school almost regularly. As a matter of fact those were the only two years she did.

Every time an epidemic of measles, or scarlet fever, or chicken pox, or mumps broke out, the doctor prescribed a series of shots to avoid the dangerous effects these childhood diseases could have on "her disease."

It made me sad not to be able to spend summers with the girls, but when we did get back together, we made up for it in spades. We didn't part for a minute and Anne often came to sleep in my bed.

At La Chèze, we took bicycle rides over the bumpy little roads where generation after generation we had barked our knees and elbows. And still did.

We went and picked watercress in the little pond at the end of the meadow, and there was always someone to slip on the damp turf the cows had trampled going to drink, and to sink to the ankles in the mud. We came back following the ditches.

Charles made giant kites: he stretched and glued butcher paper over a kind of scaffold made out of thin strips of wood that he bought from the village carpenter.

He stayed for hours, forgetting everything—including mealtimes—unwinding hundreds of yards of string and following far off in the sky the little spot that soared like a bird.

Sometimes he put the children in charge of holding the wooden handle the string was wound on. It was hard to hold, and Anne was so light she'd be lifted from the ground.

Sometimes a gust of wind, a little stronger than usual, brought the string down and pulled the kite loose. Everybody went looking for the big paper bird and usually found it panting on the top of a tree. One day it landed delicately in a furrow a peasant was plowing; the man was very surprised: "What kind of creature is that?" He must have been thinking of the Martians there was a lot of talk about at the time.

Caroline was the director for the plays the children devised. She did the casting. She was very authoritarian with her cousins and rehearsals never occurred without quarrels and some fistfights.

She contrived funny costumes and sets. Sophie always had the longest parts, maybe because she was the most talkative one in the gang. What's more, she recited them at breakneck pace. Eric, always the good guy and a little clumsy, accepted the least rewarding roles. Laurence usually played a man, and the two blond children, Anne and her cousin, Marc, moved the sets around or carried trays, but remained mute.

Zoulette played the prompter.

One time, they put on a funny play in which all the words were twisted and for a long time we'd hear sentences like, "Zounds, 'tis my zusmand," every time a husband appeared, or "Coming, mudder," every time they were called.

That summer we celebrated Anne's and Marc's wedding with great pomp. She was seven years old.

Zoulette and Caroline made a long dress out of a sheet, and a veil from a mosquito net. It was held to her head with a crown of wild grapevines.

Marc wore his father's blazer which hit his calves and a top hat that creased his ears.

The whole family, including Mamy, their great-grandmother, put on fancy clothes, extravagant hats, and grotesque finery.

Eric was the verger and walked at the head of the strange procession which bawled out Mendelssohn's wedding march.

We laughed a lot and I remember that the bride's smile particularly enchanted everyone. Anne had lost a front tooth the day before.

We spent every Christmas at Valgenceuse, Charles' family's place north of Paris. It is a very beautiful, romantic estate. The eighteenth-century park was designed by LeNotre, who designed Versailles.

I arrived just the day before and we hauled down the cartons of tinsel and balls that we kept from year to year.

We seemed to grow more demanding every Christmas, for there was never enough to dress the tree with.

Kakoze had to go with Anne and ransack the last shops in Senlis. Anne would come home delighted, waving new strings of many-colored lights.

The tree was stuck into the bottom of a big blue vase in the gallery. There was always the problem of a ladder to reach the top and hook on the star, and the problem of a multiple socket for connecting the elaborate lighting. The girls were in charge of the lower branches and fought over who would get the biggest crystal balls.

When at last the lights were plugged in and the tree sparkled, it was truly Christmas.

All the adults would leave, under one pretext or another, and shut themselves into their rooms with rolls of fancy colored paper and balls of gold string to do the giftwrapping.

We brought down the packages meant for the "big ones" and arranged them on the pool table. We opened them between dinner and midnight mass, everyone squealing and laughing, "ho-ho" and "ha-ha." Then we sat on the edge of the pool table or in those lovely Charles X chairs and totally uncomfortable banquettes. Or grandma got out her violin, Uncle David sat down at the piano, and Aunt Pauline warbled a song in her melodious, old-fashioned voice.

Around eleven o'clock grandma put on her lined boots and coaxed us to leave for the cathedral "if we want to get seats." We sang at the top of our lungs during mass to keep ourselves warm. Indeed there were some spots where the gas heat worked but we burned our heads when we stood up. And anyway seats near these sources of heat were always taken by the time we got there.

The boys' choir was something to hear, and the young soloist sang the opening of *O Lord, how deep Thy silence . . .*

too high and went off key when he attacked the second phrase and tried to link *When e'er the golden stars* to the first.

Sometimes we had fits of laughter, as you have only in places where you shouldn't, and Anne and Laurence would hide in the skirts of my coat.

After mass we went by the fish store and picked up a large tray with several dozen oysters all opened and piled precariously upon it. And if they still had a little water in the hollow of their shells when we got home it was a miracle. Then we sent the girls off to bed, but first they put a shoe in front of each fireplace. A single shoe because there were more fireplaces than they had pairs of shoes.

On Christmas morning, Zoulette kept them as long as possible in front of her own fireplace where three toys were enthroned. The first of the joyful harvest.

Then Zoulette released the girls into the hallways and there was galloping and happy screaming from room to room. Grandma's room, Kakoze's, and ours. I think Kakoze's fireplace provided the greatest delights and the best surprises.

On Christmas day, the whole Valgenceuse family poured into a beautiful house in Senlis for a gargantuan and tasty meal. The menu never varied, which was all to the good. We banished Anne's diet on such days. Her cheeks glowed with pleasure.

Two years in a row, the pond with the big linden trees all around froze for Christmas. I knocked my heel on the edge before venturing on the ice, one step at a time to the middle. And when the ice cracked slightly, a long gash would run with a muffled whistle up to the stone staircase behind me and allow me to figure how thick the ice was. Then I would wave for the children to come.

They laced their skates and came down the embankment, turning their ankles inward. First they clung to an iron chair which usually slid faster than they did, and they found themselves doing belly flops on the ice.

That Christmas, the winter of 1962, was an especially gay one for Anne. She was seven. For the first time she put on small boots with wide blades and was thrilled with all the sliding. Her very thin ankles twisted but she didn't complain. She had the amazing tenacity and will-power to follow the others without admitting to pain or fatigue.

From then until spring, incidentally, she went every week to take lessons at Molitor Skating Rink and she did very well.

When night fell, after all the sliding on the pond, she served us tea. She loved being allowed to take the initiative and quite soon, in Paris, it became her job to go and buy cigarettes and the papers.

In Grandma's fireplace that year, the girls found a puff ball table; Anne would grab the rubber bulb that guarded her goal and squeeze and squeeze the little white bulb to near exhaustion. She laughed her head off. She liked games and became unbeatable at *crapette, petits chevaux,* and "screw your buddy." She called it "get your, buddy," by the way, in an air both prudish and teasing.

The year 1963 found us often separated.

I had a lot of work to do and was frequently away. Also, Anne's disease had been stable for almost two years and I was not bothered too much. Secretly I almost dared to hope it had stopped.

It frightened Anne when I took a plane. Every time she said to Zoulette, "I hope Mother won't fall asleep in the plane, she could get lost."

When I left, she was very sad. And as the years went

by the feeling grew. She couldn't get used to these departures. For her they made no sense at all. And I regretted them more and more myself. I felt ever more deeply, year after year, that I was stealing time from her, her tremendously precious time. Our time. Together.

She'd also say to Zoulette after I left, "Do you think she'll come back? Are you sure nothing bad will happen to her? I'll pray that nothing will happen to her, come and say your prayers with me."

And sweet, precious Zoulette would do her best to reassure her.

When I got back, no matter what time it was, no matter what work she was doing, or what game she was involved in at the moment, Anne dropped everything.

She came to me and wouldn't leave me for a minute, nor budge an inch as long as I was at home. She offered to help me unpack, put my things in order, hang up my clothes. But she sensed that I preferred to do the job myself. Because I was always in a hurry. Always. What nonsense. She also brought my mail and would not interrupt me while I read it. She climbed on my bed and watched me as I went to and fro. She was happy. And she told me stories, about "Zaza," the dog that belonged to the woman downstairs, about the concierge who "yelled at" the Spanish women, about Caroline who had made a beautiful drawing for her, or about Laurence who had had to stay after school.

She started all her sentences with "You know."

Out of the blue one day, she told me, "You know, well, Laurence has been nice to me. I think she loves me. She let me borrow her eraser."

When I took a bath, I used to leave the door to my room open, so we could talk.

When I said nothing, because I was tired or in a bad mood, or preoccupied by something else, I'd hear her deep voice at regular intervals:

"Mother!"

"Yes."

"I love you."

A few minutes later:

"Mother!"

"What?"

"I love you."

When I came out of my bath, wrapped in a towel, she'd still be calling, softly:

"Mother!"

"What do you want?"

"I've got something to tell you. Come closer. Listen, closer please, I'll whisper it, it's a secret.

"?"

"I love you."

She did anything to hold on to me.

But I always had to leave. And not always as lightheartedly as I pretended.

Sometimes I canceled everything.

And nothing else existed. We were like two lovers meeting on the sly.

At the beginning of 1963, Anne stopped going to school. That made her unhappy. What else was there to do?

She couldn't help being absent all the time. She was too tired to attend all the classes or keep up with the schedule. So we found a young lady who came two or three times a week; and the rest of the time Anne had to work alone—with Zoulette's help of course—at exactly the same hours as if she were at school.

Anne had an alarm clock on her table and she began on the dot. On the dot she stopped. Even in the middle of a sentence or problem. She took a fifteen-minute break and went back to work.

She didn't know what cheating meant. We teased her and shook her up a bit, but nothing could unsettle the conscience and sense of duty of that frail little creature. We tried to get her to take things more lightly, to make them less important. But deep inside we respected and admired her will-power and the trouble she went to to follow the same path as the others.

She wanted to forget and to have the others forget that she wasn't well. And often she succeeded.

I told her things I thought would interest or amuse her about my life.

I even said sometimes:

"I'm going to tell you a secret."

She'd raise her eyebrows.

"Just for me?"

"Yes, nobody but you will know."

She was delighted and very proud.

"Not even the girls?"

"Not even the girls. Just you."

I knew that nothing, nobody, could make her talk till I released her from her pledge of secrecy.

So, some time in February of that year, I was asked to play a small part in a film. For fun I accepted, just to see. But I hadn't told a soul. I recalled the fit the family threw at my working at Chanel's; it would be worse this time. Only Anne knew.

I spent a full week in a big house on Rue de Birague. I got to the paper early so I could sneak away at noon, and hurry to join the film crew.

Invariably just as the little red light went on, when

silence was obtained and the purring of the camera followed the order for "action!" the telephone would ring and someone would be calling me from the paper.

The main scene I was in was a dinner, something that took place over the wine and the cheese. For days we ate some kind of Port Salut.

I remember how the exacting job of the scriptgirl fascinated me, how she had to restore the pieces of cheese to the condition they were in the day before, to put wine in the glasses—which emptied immediately, I must say—to ask us to drag on our cigarettes a bit more quickly, before resuming the scene.

It was an anguishing and pathetic film, having to do with suicide. However, there was an odd gaiety prevailing in that large, cold, damp, empty house. We behaved like school kids. The same jokes. The same fits of giggling.

When everyone went to see the rushes, I jumped on my Vespa and zipped down Rue de Rivoli to make another appearance at the paper.

Then I would go home and Anne would ask:

"Did you have cheese again today?"

"Why did you ask Mother that?" Laurence once said, her tone very inquisitive.

"Because." Anne answered.

"Because why?" her tone rising.

"Because," Anne repeated, enigmatically.

When the film opened, the family thought it was great.

You never can tell.

When summer vacation came, Anne learned how to swim at the resort, Le Touquet, and then the trio left for La Chèze.

Toward the end of July, I wrote from Paris to say that

I'd fly over the house in a little plane on my way to the Basque country.

Almost on schedule, after we had risen above the first foothills of Millevaches Plateau and wandered about for a while in the air, looking here for a steeple, there for a grove of chestnuts, the first thing I recognized was the big cedar sticking up from a tangle of greenery and roofs. Next the large meadow. There, squirming around on a sheet spread on the grass, little white shapes. The children.

The plane made a slight dive and, through the window, I tossed them a shower of candy. We circled several times. They all waved handkerchiefs. I saw little arms stretched out, little legs trotting about in the grass. The excitement was at its peak. Then we had to go. My heart was heavy. We were so close. And we couldn't touch, or hear, or really see one another. I had guessed and made out those little silhouettes by the color of their hair, and their dresses; and yet just barely.

It was like one of those dreams where, trying to reach something three feet away, just out of reach of your hand, you're dumbfounded to find out you can't walk.

We hadn't flown more than five minutes over the hills when suddenly I said, "Let's go back, just for a second."

We went back over the meadow.

They all were still there. The children were gathering up their candy. They raised their heads when they heard the sound of the engine again and the pilot decided to go very low this time to give them another salute.

Too low.

The alarm buzzer suddenly went off in the plane. Nothing crossed the pilot's face but he promptly pulled up on the joystick and we grazed the oaks bordering the meadow. In the plane, we didn't fully realize. But I later learned that for three days afterwards one of our audience had a bellyache.

As for the children, they remained waiting a long time in the meadow, hoping the plane would come back a third time. Then they leaped the stile—looking a little proud of themselves, a little sad, their pockets stuffed with candy.

After that I returned to Paris for the fashion shows.

A crazy and absurd time that was all the more so for us. As journalists for *Women's Wear Daily,* we had to send in our stories, articles, photographs, and sketches every evening so that they could be published the next morning in New York.

We went to as many as five or six fashion shows a day. And I—who always ended mixing things up, and very quickly too—I had great admiration for those professionals who were able to discern in the bat of an eye, as a model sped past, such and such a "new" detail, and to remember it next season! I was later to master this not so mysterious exercise.

We always had to know everything before anyone else. Our rule of the scoop was an absolute.

With most of the couturiers it was easy. With a few, not so. Obviously certain couturiers were not only closed to us but would gladly have been slammed shut on our noses had we put them there. In such cases we took the attitude that no holds were barred.

For instance, every season, about a week before the press show, a secretary from the paper was in charge of delivering a spray of flowers to the manager of a certain fashion house, and of presenting it to her personally. The manager could only be found in the workroom—the

Holy of Holies for couturiers—where the closely guarded fittings of the new designs took place.

The resourceful secretary had to get through several barriers. Forcefully she insisted that her boss, the florist, had expressly ordered her to deliver the flowers to no one but the lady in question.

Having reached her goal at last, she'd cast sidelong glances around her, as casual as could be.

The next day a sketch of one of the designs from the collection would appear. Often, by the way, of the climax, the pinnacle of the new line—the bridal dress. They'd tear their hair. They talked of leaks.

The most beautiful such scoop occurred by mere chance.

One day I was strolling nonchalantly along Avenue Georges V trying to get a look at whatever I could through the large window of a very expensive building that housed a famous couture concern; I decided on the spot not to lend myself to such a ridiculous game. I sat down on a bench in the sun and began to read.

Suddenly looking up, I saw a friend rush up to the main entrance of the forbidden establishment. I was intrigued. I knew for certain that he had no business in this sanctuary of frills: his job had nothing to do with the fashion industry.

I ran across the avenue and caught up with him under the archway.

"What are you doing here?" I said.

"Just going home," he answered, "that's all."

He lived there! In the very heart of the couturier's establishment. The only apartment in the building that wasn't part of it. All the windows overlooked the workshops that opened onto the big courtyard.

This apartment, incidentally, was a strange one, out-of-date and full of charm. Nothing seemed to have been changed for fifty years. It looked as if no one had ever moved the furniture or shifted an object. Nothing had been touched for ages, not even with a feather duster.

On that particular day there was a delicious smell of beef stew in the air; I shared the meal with my friends.

Of course I told them all about my own special interest in the view I got of the ant's nest with its plying of the needle, the use of the scissors and the iron, the pinning of clothes on wooden dummies or putting them on hangers. This amused them and they invited me to stay as long as I liked.

In two hours I learned enough to fill a double-page spread in the next morning's paper with sketches and details. And at the couturier's they called us pirates and they thought the leaks were now becoming serious, really disturbing.

When I told this to Anne, she said, "That's not fair."

I left for Corsica to do a series of articles.

For ten days, I scoured the island with a photographer from Ajaccio. Toussaint was a round little man, very cheerful, up to my shoulder. He drove at full tilt, singing *L'Ajaccienne;* his powerful voice hardly carried over the rattling of his old jalopy. We went from one house to another, two days here, one hour there.

We visited every "interesting" person from north to south, from the famous French poetess Louise de Vilmorin to Tino Rossi, the heart throb singer who is second only to Napoleon in Corsica.

The most curious visit we paid—a strange and intriguing one—was at Leonor Fini's. She lived in an ancient monastery whose Franciscan monks, legend has it, were pirate-monks.

To reach this monastery, rather than climb as is usually the case, you have to leave your car on the side of a little road, walk a half hour down a narrow stone path, turning your ankles on the loose stones.

Or you can arrive by sea.

Leonor Fini, dramatic, superb, wrapped in an immense blood-red shawl, came out of the chapter house to greet us. She showed us a few cells she had furnished without fuss and where she painted. There were roots of strange shapes strewn about, bizarre shells, stones, dried flowers.

In every opening, huge Siamese cats would suddenly appear, or they'd go by, silent and proud. A dozen or more of these sumptuous pussycats wandered the monastery. I knew that Leonor Fini adored them and I noticed how she herself looked so like a cat. Her look. Her gestures.

The violent crash of the sea against the rocks reverberated through the vaults.

Afterwards she took us to see the monks' graveyard. She had opened very ancient tombs and put candles in the skulls. I noticed that Toussaint kept crossing himself the whole time.

Bones were so arranged that they looked like modern sculptures. Toussaint perspired in terror.

He wanted to leave right away. But that's where he made his best pictures. Going up the path, he said to me, "You're something, you know funny people . . ." Later I learned that the municipality of Nonza got upset and asked the lady of the monastery to please put things back where they belonged, the skulls under the tombstones, and not to touch the cemetery again, though it was no longer consecrated.

The girls loved that story. Anne said, "Poor thing, she'll end up in hell."

I brought back Corsican "specialties" for the children. Minuscule keychain pistols that exploded with an infernal racket; these I gave to the girls. Little switchblades for my nephews. Five minutes later, Eric cut himself and Caroline punctured her hand.

The family bawled me out. That was normal. Somebody threw all my nice little gifts into the pond. But my father sneaked out one of the knives, and he carries it in his pocket to this day.

That year, Anne was flower girl in a wedding that took place in Reims cathedral. A big event for her.

Up to the last minute we shuddered at the idea that Anne would be too tired to attend. We couldn't stand disappointing her. It had happened once before when she couldn't accompany her sisters. This time it was her turn. With her dear little Marc. And it was all so much fun. The night spent in a hotel. The procession. She was so dignified going down the spectacular nave, ahead of the bridal couple on Marc's arm.

Hand in hand they passed the plate. Many pictures were taken. She was pale and romantic. And so pretty. Mademoiselle Mayne had made her dress. Mademoiselle Mayne was the seamstress in Chamboulive. We called her our local Coco Chanel. She lived in a very ancient house on the edge of town, on the road that goes down the hill behind the church. She went out no more than twice a day. Early in the morning to go to mass and in the afternoon to fetch her milk.

Three stone steps, well rounded by use, led to her

heavy wooden front door. Then one step down into a long, low, dark room where she plied her needle and lived. A wood stove, a pot always simmering on it, provided a little heat. A rather sour smell filled the air. Forever the same smell. A yellow cat sat on the table.

The *demoiselle* seamstress never changed. No matter the year, no matter the season, you found her with the same face, as pale as her fragile smile. No one knew how old she was. Her hair, tight and perched high in a chignon, was always the same black. A black crocheted shawl, half jacket, half cape, wrapped around her shoulders snugly. She raised it over her head to go to church when it was cool, or to go for her milk.

Nothing surprised her.

All year she made blouses with round collars and skirts with four panels that came well below the knees, but when we came on vacation we could ask her to make any silly thing and she would eagerly execute it, and to perfection.

I suspect that our bermuda shorts, which unzipped in front, our skirts to mid-thigh, and our bare backs must have provided a happy change for her.

The fittings took place in the next room. The room sloped so steeply and was so slippery and highly waxed that it was dangerous. Moreover she had this timid way of "suggesting," please, that we put on paper slippers to slide around on when we were in this room. Several windows were walled up. It was cold undressing.

The clothes she was working on at the time were carefully laid out on the puffy eiderdown that covered Mademoiselle Mayne's very high bed. Fittings went on in front of the mirror door of a heavy wooden wardrobe.

Whenever we got ready to go she pulled a little metal

box out from behind her button boxes, and offered us gum drops. She insisted that we take two, shaking the box and saying, singsong fashion, hopping each syllable, "Go on, it won't hurt you, go on now." Anne didn't like candy and she would politely refuse. Once. Twice. Then, daring not say why she didn't care for one, she would whisper, "I'm not hungry."

The prettiest house on the village square, and also the most ramshackle, right across from the wide steps of the church, was the most mysterious.

A lady had lived there alone, for so long a time that no one knew how long it was. Her bent silhouette, properly hatted, was visible only for a moment, as she crossed the road between her house and the church.

That's where she spent most of her time, arranging the altar flowers, watching every entrance and exit, calling the kids to task for roughhousing during the services, and being a general pain in the neck for Reverend Father.

The pious lady spent all her money making improvements in the beautiful structure that overshadowed her house. We had a grudge against her for destroying bit by bit all the folklore of our childhood—like the time she had electric bells installed in the church.

We all yearned for the huge ropes that hung in the middle of the church, which three kids could cling to and pull with their slender arms and be swept up like disjointed puppets when the deep bass bell began to ring.

People said that Mme de . . . had once been very beautiful with the coppery hair of a lioness. That she had married a charming man whom the Spanish flu had "taken away" a week after the wedding. So she had buried herself behind the closed shutters for many long years and nobody had entered the lovely house since. It was a sad story, a sad life. Nobody likes sad stories that last a lifetime.

But then we longed to know what it was like behind those macramé curtains, and under that large slate roof that nobody had climbed since the beginning of the century.

In January 1964, when she was nine, Anne began her vomiting. She had a fever. The tests were bad. She began a series of shots, the only result of which was to make her cry every time the nurse appeared with the large syringe in her hand. Anne hid her face in Zoulette's apron and clung to it with all her might. She didn't flinch all the time the big needle was being stuck into her buttock, a buttock no bigger than an apple. Afterwards, the nurse would say, "Now tell the truth, it didn't hurt much, did it?" Not so sure, Anne pouted and smiled politely.

We decided to go to the hospital.

Professor Z's ward had just been transferred from Enfants Malades to Hérold. This hospital was at the very edge of Paris. At the very edge of the world, to us.

Hérold was old and grimmer than Enfants Malades. However the children's section had recently been redone and repainted to make it more attractive.

The doctors and nurses greeted Anne so nicely, that morning of January 13, that she was all smiles as I left with Zoulette.

She went through transfusions, and perfusions. The nurse remembered that she was left-handed and immobilized her right arm.

When I went back the next day, I found Anne sad and silent. "Am I going home today?" she asked.

Of course we had told her "one or two days" when we arrived. So I said "tomorrow," unable to add "maybe." Her eyes were clouded with tears. She turned her head on the pillow and said nothing. Neither did I. I didn't know what to say. I hated lying to her.

The next day I found her bathed in tears. Not a sob. Not a murmur. Not a word of protest. Not a groan. Nothing but this distressing sadness. The sadness of an adult.

"I've never seen the likes," the nurse said. "She refuses to take any nourishment. She cries in silence. She never complains. There's nothing we can do to entertain her. Everybody in the ward is so sorry."

I tried to reason with Anne, to explain to her. She listened nicely. But I sensed a really amazing determination in her eyes. Something completely new. I was so upset I could hardly keep back my tears.

Over and over again she'd say softly, "I want to go home."

And she'd add, "Why am I sick?" It was a question without an answer.

At the end of the fourth day, it was still the same. Anne's attitude had not changed. The doctor was really moved now and decided to let her go home.

Nanou had won.

It was Thursday. Zoulette was out.

I smuggled Anne into the house. She was smiling. Now and then in the car she gave me a little nudge with her elbow.

"You're not mad at me, are you, Mother?"

I stopped the car and kissed her voraciously.

When we got home, she devoured a chicken thigh with French fries, then sneaked into her bed, very happy, and said:

"I'm going to scare Zoulette when she gets back."

When Zoulette came in, she let out her "ho-hos" and ha-has" of joy and surprise.

The next day the doctor called to say that the disease had indeed started again. "It's entering a new stage of development." It had these periods of regression. Then just as we took heart it would suddenly flare up again in some new part of her body. The doctor said he would like to show Anne to a group of professors, pediatricians, and specialists who were particularly interested in the disease and whose advice he wanted to have.

We made an appointment for February 19 at Hérold hospital. We arrived early, Zoulette, Anne, and I. Everybody in the ward was ready.

As we waited for all the chief doctors to get there, we were taken on a tour of the preemies in their incubators. Anne couldn't believe her eyes when she saw the miniature size of these bits of humanity lying in their glass boxes.

The babies made short, jerky movements with their skinny little arms, and opened and closed their fingers like sea anemones.

Anne was fascinated and wanted to know how they ate, how they breathed, and (in a low voice) how they went poopoo.

At last we were told that everybody was coming. We were led into a large room. At one end was a row of chairs behind a long table, and other rows of chairs were arranged in semicircles. It must have been a kind of lecture hall where courses were given.

One by one, doctors, professors, interns, externs, nurses, assistants, and other people, all in white smocks, entered. I counted twenty-two of them.

The oldest was Professor Debré. He came up to us to

say hello and nicely pinched Anne's cheek. He then sat down at the center of the row behind the table. Professor Z and his assistants surrounded him. The others took their places in the rows of chairs.

Zoulette, Anne, and I were in the first row. There was silence. Anne was a little anxious. I could see she wasn't missing a thing. Warily she watched the strange goings-on. She responded to the smiles with a somewhat twisted smile of her own.

Professor Z stood up and read a report concerning Anne's disease. It lasted for more than fifty minutes. From time to time Professor Debré raised a question, asking for details. I noticed how tense and attentive he was. His deep intelligent look seemed to be sorting things out from all the impressive language.

When the reading was over, nobody made a move until Debré said he wanted to see Anne. They had her sit on the table and all the white smocks surrounded her. She was asked to remove her dress. She did this right away. She, who showed such delicacy where emotions were concerned, had no notion of physical modesty. To undress, to appear completely nude, was a matter of total indifference to her. It was one of those things one has to do. So she did it. Quite naturally.

The Professor's eyes ran lightly over the slight body and paused attentively on Anne's face, and on that red spot the shape of a butterfly which had reappeared on the cheekbones. He said, "You're very pretty."

That's all he said. His face showed a great kindness. A great inner calm. He left, followed at a respectful distance by the whole group.

On the way home, Anne asked me: "What was all that for?"

"To prove that you're all right. And that you're beautiful," I answered.

And she said, "You're nice, Mother. I love you."

A few days later they gave me the conclusion these distinguished gentlemen had reached. They were all of the opinion that the dosage of Cortancyl should be increased. Some were pessimistic about the future, especially the youngest among them. Others were more optimistic. They advised that a renal biopsy be made—that is, a piece of tissue removed from the kidneys; this would enable confirmation of the diagnosis and perhaps also better indicate the therapy. Others thought that such an operation was a waste of time. They discussed it. They decided to wait, maybe even to give it up.

I didn't tell Anne, of course. We dropped the subject. For eighteen months.

I entered a period of anguish and of a frantic drive to please Anne. To shower her with everything. To entertain her. To see her happy. To see her laugh. To see her live.

We had her portrait done. I took her to lunch at the Pub Renault. And to the Chinese restaurant. I took her to the movies, *A Mad, Mad, Mad, Mad World, Tintin and the Blue Oranges, Merlin the Magician.* She saw the ballet *Cinderella.* I rented a television set.

She was very tired. Everything tired her. But she was happy. That's what mattered. She was sore everywhere: headaches, bellyaches, knee aches, nausea. She tried so hard. All the time. Because happiness was much more important than pain. Because she wanted to see things. To participate. To live. She fought.

In the morning she'd stand in front of a mirror to see if she "looked good." No. She didn't look good. Too bad.

Nothing in the world could have made her miss her sittings at the painter's, in Montmartre, in narrow Rue Tholozé, so steep that we had to attack it from a staircase above. It didn't take long but I saw the circles forming under her eyes.

Sometimes there was a long line in front of a movie theater. She wanted to wait. I tried to dissuade her. No. No. No.

Once, we had waited a long time, standing up at the Pub to have seats on the imitation leather banquettes. She had leaned against a wooden column. I watched her thin face becoming even more angular.

Zoulette looked at me, worried. I asked Anne, "Are you tired?" "No. Why?"

"Nothing. Just asking."

I showed her a fat lady who was gorging herself with whipped cream. "Ugh," said Anne laughing.

Finally we were seated. She ordered a chocolate sundae. Slowly, delicately, she pushed the whipped cream to the side and nibbled two small spoonfuls of chocolate ice cream. Then she put down her spoon.

"I'm not hungry anymore. Sorry."

"We'll give it to the fat lady. OK?"

We pirouetted. We played games. Our complicity increased daily.

She had been dazzled by the ballet *Cinderella.*

A lovely show for little girls.

Some time afterwards, I met Geraldine Chaplin, who danced in *Cinderella.* When I got home I told Anne about having seen one of the dancers in *Cinderella.* Her eyes sparkled.

"Mother, I've got something to ask you," she said after

a few moments. "Do you think I could take up dancing?"

"Why not?"

It was very seldom she asked for anything.

I loved it when she felt like doing this or that. When she wanted nothing it meant that she wasn't feeling well.

We found a dancing school near the house. I bought her leotards and ballet shoes and she placed them in a little Air-France bag.

Alas, she took only a few lessons. It was hard for her to follow. Too tiring for her. We had to give it up. Yet she loved it. She was terribly sorry, but she said, "Never mind, I'll do something else."

She soon got over things. Happily. She always looked for some consolation in any disappointment.

At that time Laurence, who was only eleven months older than Anne, was four grades ahead of her. It was very important that Anne do something her sisters didn't do. There had been dancing, but we had to give that up. Sports were almost out of the question . . .

Still, three summers in a row, Laurence first had a donkey at La Chèze, then a big horse called Bucephalus. Laurence was entirely in charge of them, she petted them, groomed them, even slept with them sometimes. She built an obstacle course for herself and jumped and galloped in the meadows. Anne followed her sister, dragged in bales of straw, helped her prepare the stall, raised a corner of the saddle to hoist her onto Bucephalus.

Laurence issued orders that brooked no argument. She was indeed the most competent of the gang and took some advantage of it.

The reward was a horseback ride. But not too long a one, not to tire the dear Bucephalus—who had the softest vacation of his horse-life at our place.

When the moment came for the ride, often late in the afternoon to avoid the heat, Anne crammed her cap on her blond head, put one foot into Laurence's cupped hands. "No, not like that," Laurence would shout, "Faster, grrr! Clumsy thing! Get going! Oo-la-la! Okay, that's good!" It was good. Then you heard, "Your wrists! Your heels!" Laurence held the lead line and Anne went proudly down the road. Laurence always stormed about but she was never careless. She knew her little sister wasn't to fall. That that would have been dangerous for her.

The two big ones were very gifted in drawing, Anne not at all.

On the other hand, she was quick at card games. She caught on right away and would win almost every time.

One day, when we were talking about what the girls would do when they "grew up," Caroline said, "I'll be a couturier and I'll design all the collections." Laurence said, "I'll ride in the equestrian competition at the next Olympics." Anne said, "I'll be a card player."

We decided she'd clean up at the Monte-Carlo and Deauville casinos, that she'd certainly be the wealthiest of us all, and in the end the whole family would sponge off her.

Anne was delighted.

Neither of the two big ones played a musical instrument. They just scratched a little at the guitar. We decided that Anne would take piano.

We moved the old black rosewood upright, with the copper candlesticks on either side of the keyboard, out of their great-grandmother's place where it was never used. My whole childhood I had heard my aunts hammering on it and joining in a chorus of "When Salome appeared without her ve-ils . . . In front of Herod she would we-ar . . . All the perfumes of Ju-de-a on her golden flesh and in her ha-ir . . ."

When they reached the final stanza, my brother and I would howl with them:

" . . . *And the tyrant fe-ll, under her voluptuous spe-ll.*"

My grandmother was horrified.

There was another song I remember. It was very fast and went:

"When you grow old darling Chee-chee
You'll bow your head low darling Chee-chee
If I knew then what I know now, aaaaaaah . . .

We exhaled that "aaaah" with every ounce of strength in our lungs. At that point Mamy really tried to get mad. To make us shut up. "All that noise. Think of the neighbors."

The poor dear hadn't much authority and we resumed all the louder:

". . . *Aaaaah, la bella Catharineta!*"

Then usually we heard the neighbor, exasperated, rap on the wall, and Mamy would say, shrugging her shoulders, "See, now see what you've done? I told you."

Anne was much more modest. So much so that she would never play in front of us. I think she was afraid of Laurence teasing her, but also Marc played so well. Anyway it didn't matter.

Zoulette said that she was doing her scales very conscientiously when no one was around, when everyone was out of the house.

At the end of the year, there was a display of Japanese mechanical men in a department store and everybody gave them to Anne. She would wind them all up at the same time in her room, five or six at once:

The little fellow who dipped a ring into a bucket, brought it up close to his mouth and blew soap bubbles that danced for a while in the light of the room, then burst as they landed delicately on the furniture;

the cook who fried an egg in a skillet and, with a flick of the wrist, turned it over;

the businessman-bear seated behind his desk, who picked up the telephone when it rang and took notes, the receiver stuck to his ear;

and the hobo who emptied his bottle of red, while hanging onto a lamppost.

It was wonderful, all that agitation.

At that time, too, I went to interview the singer, Juliette Greco.

She owns a marvelous collection of antique automatons. They're all on the floor in her room, and their expressions are so real it's upsetting, all standing on the Aubusson rug, as are the lamps, the candlesticks, and all the objects surrounding the large bed that is only the thickness of a single mattress.

When she entered her room, Greco jostled a flower: "I'm sorry, rose," she said, then she wound up her mechanical men and addressed them: "Dear objects, I love you so tenderly, I collect you with passion, with love. But I'm not hooked on you. I'm hopeless, don't you think?"

The dark-haired little man in dinner jacket lights a cigar. He takes a puff, inhales, throws his head back slightly. In his eyes there is an expression of undefinable, voluptuous pleasure.

The dreaming Pierrot, under his wide, white satin hat, writes at a little old desk. A kerosene lamp lights his pen. Now and then he raises his head, shakes it slowly as if he were looking for inspiration, then he lowers his chin and falls asleep.

In the room there were also several portraits of Juliette Greco by Fujita, Umbłot, and others. The City of Paris had recently purchased one of them, which made Juliette say, with a big laugh, "Greco! At the Louvre!"

I had promised Anne to take her to see the collection. Some day.

She was feeling better.

So, once more, we had some time. Time to live. To speak of the future. To make plans.

The state of emergency had vanished.

And I didn't keep my promise.

But I took the trio to hear the Beatles at the Palais des Sports. I knew it was a major undertaking and I was careful to reserve seats near an exit. One never knows. But the performance was worth the effort and we had agreed, the two older girls and I, that in case the expression "bring down the house" were literally and physically put into execution we'd make a protective wedge with our bodies and put Anne in the middle in our escape.

It was cold and the seats were hard, but after a short while we had forgotten about all that. We were anesthetized by the music and the crazy noise from all kinds of whistling, howling, moaning. Our seats shook and vibrated with the frantic stomping of feet set up by the horde of fans.

I watched the girls on the sly; not one of them turned a hair. Modesty. Timidity. In any case, no hysteria. I preferred that. Just their tense expressions, eyes slightly creased shut, mouths half-opened in a kind of smile, and also a finger, a knee or the tip of a foot moving, keeping the beat, letting you guess their passionate interest.

From time to time, when the P.A. reached a paroxysm of violence, Anne frowned a little and stopped her ears.

It was a "super" performance. The girls were delighted. Anne dragged a little going home, it's true, but she had a good reason. She'd had such fun.

She was much better.

So much so that she went back to classes at Dupanloup for a few months.

She worked very hard and often got a prize. Whenever she came home proudly sporting her decoration on her blue coat, we said, "Hail to the General."

She wrote things in her tablet, such as: "I worked well in school today. I'm pleased."

She began to work on absurd little math problems involving faucets and railroads.

The poor thing understood not a bit of it; she perspired; she was in despair facing all those numbers. She wrote slantwise in the margin: "Do I put it down under the 4 or under the 0?"

Zoulette showed it to me in secret. I wonder if we're going to go on loading our kids with bullshit like this forever. Probably so.

Although I tried to explain to Anne that it didn't matter in the least, that it was all totally useless, she didn't believe me. Of course she didn't. And I didn't insist.

When Zoulette had to go away on vacation, Anne was desperate. She didn't show it, but in her tablet we found things like: "Zoulette, I love you and I'm sad you're leaving for Binic. Think of me and how you made me do my homework," or, "Zoulette, pray for me and my arithmetic."

Sometimes she was very funny. She'd make a pun and burst out laughing, throwing her head back.

One day, during lunch, Caroline and Laurence were looking for the names of the muscles of the human body.

"There are the biceps," said Caroline.

"And the triceps too," said Laurence.

"And the quadruple sex too," said Anne.

That year we moved to larger quarters.

We couldn't stand the irritating lack of space of the apartment any longer—standing in line to take a bath and unfolding a bed every night in the drawing room.

It took us more than a year to unpack the piles of crates in the new one. We never had time. We didn't care much either. And the girls played hide and seek among them.

On June 11, 1965, a consultation took place at Enfants Malades with five great specialists, one of them American. They discussed the matter and decided to take a kidney smear. The American specialist said that two cases of the disease were reported in America. Two adolescents on whom they have already done several biopsies. Two cases they still hoped to cure.

The day of the operation was set: September 20. Anne was ten.

The summer was spent biking, swimming in the pond at Mérignac, galloping around on a donkey, and pulling each other's hair.

Once in a while Zoulette took Anne to "confession" and I always wondered what in the world either could have to reproach herself for.

I came to see them one weekend in a car that was all electric gadgets.

The children spent their time raising and lowering the windows, putting the roof up and down, pushing all the buttons, making everything go.

One day, I piled all of them in to go to the pond. There, everybody undressed and we put the clothes in the trunk. I removed the keys from the dashboard, threw them in my basket, put the basket in the trunk, and slammed the lid.

And there we were in our bathing suits standing around our beautiful, hermetically sealed car. La Chèze was ten miles away, and a tiny village was two.

Anne got upset.

So I decided to go, on foot of course, along the little road that wriggled its way between chestnut trees up to the village.

Eric went with me.

I was barefoot and in a bikini.

On entering the village I didn't know where to put the bit of a towel I had: around my hips or over my shoulders, in front or behind? I decided in favor of in front. People gave us funny looks. I asked if there was a garage. They pointed to a small shed. There, a man was sprawled under a light truck.

"Sir," Eric shouted, "sir."

The man was hammering and didn't hear. Eric pulled at his pants.

"What do you want?" said the man, slipping like a frog from under the vehicle.

I explained that our car was locked with the keys inside. It was me he listened to but he looked at Eric. Obviously he was as embarrassed by my apparel as I was.

"But then," he said after a while, "how come you got it locked with the keys inside?"

A logical question.

"Because it's automatic," I said sheepishly.

"Don't know nothing about stuff like that," he grumbled, shaking his head.

He went and rummaged around under his workbench and came back with a set of keys (none of which matched the one we needed) as well as a master key and a monkey wrench.

Without a word, he got into his truck and made a sign for us to climb in. We returned to the side of the pond. We fiddled around with all the locks. In vain.

So we cut a piece out of the roof. Just enough for Eric to sneak first his head and then himself inside the car. He crawled over the rear seat and, nobody knows how, got inside the trunk where he recovered the damn keys.

Shrugging his shoulders, the man went back to his little village of normal people. Far from those half-naked nuts fidgeting around a strongbox they used as a car.

On September 19, Zoulette took Anne to mass and played *crapette* with her after lunch.

At five, I took her to the clinic.

I had explained to her a few days before that she would be operated on. That she'd receive a shot to put her to sleep. That we were not going to the hospital but to a clinic where she'd have a big bed in a large room of her own. What is more, there'd be a bed for me too and every night I'd come to have dinner and sleep over with her.

This prospect seemed delightful:

"We're going to have fun," she said. "You'll lock the door so they'll leave the two of us alone. We'll play games and we'll turn the lights out very late."

Then, with her conspiratorial air, she added, "You won't tell the girls, huh? Will you?"

"No, my little Zouzou."

There I go deceiving her again, I said to myself, cheating. But what else could I do?

We adults can do anything to children. We give them no choice. And they accept anything from us, blindly, with a total trust that should leave us a bad conscience. It's bothering, a bad conscience, but how easily one adapts to it!

How often I thought of that, going through hospital wards. How many times I wished I could take people by the hand, and lead them to the hospital ward. "Open your eyes and look. You'll find here, or any other place where children are suffering, all the courage and resignation in the world. If you come across a sad look, you won't forget it, but you'll never hear a child uttering a reproach or a complaint."

In illness children are admirable. Exemplary. Overwhelming.

Anne packed some copies of *Tintin* and *Astérix* in her suitcase, some playing cards, the *petits chevaux* game, a box of pearls. Before leaving, she cut a lock of her hair and gave it to Zoulette; Zoulette put it in a locket. Anne said, "Zoulette, your eyes are red. Don't be sad, I'm going to have fun with Mother."

When we arrived at the clinic, a nun installed us in a lovely, bright room. Anne thought the beds were good. We played all kinds of games all evening. Anne won every time. She laughed. She was delighted.

For dinner they brought her only bouillon and a compote. Then they made my bed next to hers. We chatted for a moment in the dark. She was the one to press the pear-shaped switch to put out the light.

In the dark I wondered if perhaps I should ask that the operation be performed the day after tomorrow, not tomorrow, so we'd have another long day and another night to play and laugh, the two of us. Uppermost in my mind was the idea that this operation was not necessary, that its only purpose would be to confirm what we already knew. . . .

And then the contradictory thoughts raced through my mind; back and forth the arguments went. It was better to get it over with. But why make Anne suffer yet again? If only it could help in some way, cure her. Maybe? Yes, the doctors were right; this would enlighten them. We were going to find out precisely what shape the kidneys were in. Yet Professor Z wasn't enthusiastic about the operation. . . . He was so nice. He didn't like to cause Anne pain. He hated to see children suffer. He loved them so. It was too bad he didn't have any of his own. How sad that Anne couldn't receive a kidney transplant. I knew perfectly well it was impossible; the disease would settle in the new one right away. What could we do?

I had to sleep and be cheerful tomorrow, and tough. Anne was sleeping quietly. I heard her soft and regular breathing. It was good, the two of us together.

The nun woke us up at six-thirty. They brought me coffee. I'd have preferred tea. It agrees with me early in the morning.

I monkeyed around getting dressed in the room. Anne laughed. Then they came to get Anne ready. They painted her body all over with iodine.

She gave me a funny and disgusted look.

Then they gave her a first shot to make her drowsy. They asked her to stay quietly lying down, and they asked me not to talk to her.

We stayed, hand in hand, for almost two hours, without saying a word. Now and then Anne would raise her large eyelids, her look a little vague. She was half asleep. I gave her hand a gentle squeeze.

A friend came to wait with me. She's a friend who shows up only when she's welcome. A rare and precious thing. Her instinct and intuition are unbelievable. Almost frightening, she says. I was not surprised that she came that morning.

At 11:20 they took Anne away on a cart.

I smoked. I read the paper. I remembered nothing about it. I tried not to think. To kill time, as the saying goes.

At one o'clock they brought Anne back, wrapped in a sheet. She was ashen. A tube stuck out of her mouth. They turned her on her side. And I waited. I waited for the pink to return to her cheeks. For her to wake up. They came to put her "into perfusion."

She awoke very soon. And tried to move. Her face was all puckered up.

"It hurts," she said under her breath.

"It will stop, Nanou, I'm here."

I looked at this little body, so thin and frail, it hardly made a bump under the sheet.

"I'm thirsty," she whispered.

I tried to lift her gently, as gently as possible. She was sore all over. But she forced a smile.

The whole afternoon, the whole night were spent this way.

"Mother, it hurts."

She didn't know how to turn over, how to rest, how to sleep.

At the crack of dawn, sleep overwhelmed me. I dozed off and her feeble voice awoke me. I felt as if I had slept for hours. But it was only a few minutes—one or two maybe.

"I'm sorry, Mother, but . . . it hurts."

I lifted up the sheet. A big bandage encased her whole body. It would be two days before I found out just how much it must have hurt—a long gash that almost completely encircled her tiny frame.

The next day, every time someone knocked on the door to bring flowers or gifts, Anne said, "How nice of them to think of me." Then she'd close her eyes and wait patiently.

Three days later we resumed our game of *crapette.*

The fourth day we went back home.

At home her cousin Marc spent the afternoons playing with Anne.

She spent the night in my bed.

October 2, I went with Anne to see Professor Z. I found him very pessimistic.

The operation confirmed the diagnosis and revealed a serious renal lesion.

He explained that a kidney lesion never recedes. That whatever harm is done is done, because the destroyed cells do not reconstitute themselves. That the thing to do now was to stop the destruction. After all, one could live with a lesion in the kidneys.

I mentioned an artificial kidney. He appeared skeptical.

I took Anne to see the movie *Fantastic Journey.*

Ten days later, on October 16, I left for the United States. I took the slides with me. Precious and microscopic testimony of the biopsy. I had to show them to the American specialist in New York.

I remember how struck I was by the modernity, the comfort, the light of that immense hospital in the Bronx.

Everything was automatic, gleaming, luxurious there. Hadn't the chief at the paper so nicely asked me, and how many times urged me, invited me even, to take Anne to America, to this place. I had always refused, thinking that her solitude and distress would be even greater in a place where she would not understand the language. Also, to make such a trip just to go into a hospital—as attractive as it might be—it was too sad. What's more I don't think it would have changed a thing. But when I thought of our old Europe, with its gray hospitals, their decrepit walls and dim corridors, their stink even, I was heartbroken.

The nurses, spotless in their starched, light blue caps, were friendly and efficient.

I called ahead to make an appointment with the great doctor who was the head of the hospital. They put me through in a few seconds. He gave me an appointment right away, and when I arrived at the hospital I was led in to him immediately.

The doctor told me that very thorough research on this disease was going on in America, that he was in direct contact with the Paris doctors and that, if any new treatment was discovered, he would instantly inform his colleagues. He also said that Anne was in the hands of the most competent doctors in Europe and that everything that could have been done up to now had been done.

He spoke slowly, searching for the simplest words he could find. I noticed how medical terminology, with its Greek and Latin roots, is identical in all languages.

He told me about the two cases he was treating here, and how he hoped for a cure.

Then a blond nurse called him away. He apologized and accompanied me to the elevator door.

"Don't worry and take care," he said, giving me a friendly tap on the shoulder.

In the taxi back, past the outskirts of Harlem, I watched a group of black youngsters playing ball in an empty lot inside a high wire fence.

It reminded me of *West Side Story.* Not long before I had taken the three girls to see the film. I had already seen it myself and I remembered only its beauty. I had forgotten the violence.

Toward the middle of the film I had wanted to take the girls out, but they were determined to stay. I sensed that they were being overwhelmed and that bothered me. I thought they'd have nightmares, that they'd be frightened and sad.

All of which did indeed happen. But, long afterwards, they said that it had been the most beautiful movie they'd ever seen. A long time afterwards, because, as we left the theater, the four of us, by tacit agreement, decided not to tell anyone that we had seen *West Side Story.*

I made up my mind to telephone them. Anne's throaty voice would be good to hear.

Suddenly I was washed by a sense of serenity. I was sure that Anne would be cured. It was obvious that a treatment would be found, a remedy, a means. Here, where so much research was going on.

When I got back to Paris, I found Anne very tired. She had pains in one leg and limped slightly. She had a high count of albumin and urea in the urine. Her Cortancyl dosage was increased.

Her cheeks, her belly, her legs began to swell. Her skin was distended, here and there cracked, the big scar stretched and enlarged. She loved salt. It was absolutely forbidden her. Scrupulously she followed her diet. Every morning Zoulette filled one of her pillboxes with all the medicine she was supposed to take that day. She never forgot. She never made a mistake.

Every time I got back from a trip, I'd bring—among other things, of course—a pillbox.

She had a whole collection of them. In leather, in porcelain, in metal. A red one, a green one, a white one. She matched them to her dress, or to her mood. When she was invited somewhere, she always took the same one, with a turquoise mounted on the lid.

The doctor said she should get a lot of rest. That she shouldn't go to school for the time being. Anne received a big card with a drawing of the Virgin and Child.

Inside the card, were many little pieces of paper signed by all her classmates at the convent school.

There were things written like:

"I hope you'll be feeling better soon."

"I hope you'll be coming back to class soon."

"I hope you're not too bored at home."

"I hope that you'll come back at Easter."

There were twenty-eight of them . . . Claire, Véronique, Sabine, Delphine, Nathalie . . . and almost as many different spellings for "hope":

The last of them said:

"I'm sad that you don't come to school no more I want you to got better."

Anne was very touched.

In early November there was a lot of talk about *Viva Maria.* The girls looked at the pictures of those "*petites Parisiennes*" in their crinoline dresses. They waited impatiently for the film to open.

I had an article to do on Brigitte Bardot.

Timidly, Anne asked, "Can I come with you?"

"Another time. Not this time. I promise."

Another promise I didn't keep. Why? I don't know really. It would have been easy. Every time I wanted such a thing, anytime I asked if I could bring her, it never posed a problem. But I very seldom spoke about Anne. Through modesty, timidity, out of fear of boring people —I don't know why. I think it was partly for fear that people would look on her as a girl apart, someone strange because of all the special treatment she received. And then I always thought there'd be another time, another chance, another opportunity, another occasion, when in fact I ought not to have let a single one slip by.

I often think of that. I regret it.

"So don't forget to bring home an autograph," said Anne.

I brought three of them. One for each. Some nice words in Brigitte's large handwriting on the back of each picture.

At that time, there was a fawn living on Rue Decamps near our house. Orphaned at the start of the hunting season, he had been harbored by some people in their country house where he lived for several days keeping warm in the kitchen.

When it came time to return to Paris, the cook had become so fond of the little creature that she flatly refused to part from it.

So she took the fawn to Paris.

One morning, Kakoze came looking for the girls to take them to see our strange and charming neighbor. The little deer continued to live in the kitchen where the kind woman had put down a rug so that he wouldn't skid on his delicate hooves. For breakfast he drank chocolate milk from a bottle. He slept in her room. When she went shopping she took him with her on a leash. He jumped gracefully on and off the elevator and trotted along the asphalt pavement. Getting over curbs at first presented difficulties. Bambi would miscalculate his leap and find himself off balance on his high wide-apart legs. In the afternoon he went for walks in the Bois de Boulogne.

He soon became very popular in the neighborhood.

Alas, Bambi grew up. He was no longer able to get into an elevator. It was out of the question to have him climb stairs. He bumped into furniture and knocked everything about.

So he was returned to his forest.

"He won't get any more chocolate milk," Anne said. "What will happen to him now?"

In January 1966, it was very cold.

Anne became even more swollen. She was entirely changed. Her cheeks were enormous. Her eyes, her bit of a nose, her mouth seemed shrunken, too small for her gross new face—this face whose perfect balance was now broken. We were all saddened. We didn't let it show. And we did everything we could to distract Anne, to make her forget this absurd and cruel change.

Sometimes we surprised her, up on her tiptoes looking sadly at herself in the mirror. I'd take her in my arms.

She'd say, "I don't care, you know." But I knew she did care.

She saw *L'Aiglon* on the stage. She also saw *Peter Pan, Fantomas Gone Wild, Mary Poppins, Twenty Thousand Leagues under the Sea.* She loved movies.

In February I took Caroline and Laurence to a winter resort. I had hoped to take Anne too. But the doctor firmly advised against it. "I promise to take you next year," I said.

"That's all right. While you're gone I'll go roller skating in the Trocadéro."

How easy everything was with her.

It was on the esplanade of the Trocadéro one day that a bunch of schoolgirls hailed Anne: "Hey, Fatty, what're you doing out of school?"

Anne blushed. Poor Zouk, so good! Why did such things have to happen? . . .

Zoulette had tears in her eyes telling me about it. I choked with anger. I hollered, "They are dirty little bitches, dumb and mean."

Then I heard Anne's gruff voice, softly saying:

"It's not their fault. They didn't know."

The first morning, on a very gentle slope, Caroline broke her leg.

While the doctor was setting her fracture, I took her pulse. Then I brought her back to the chalet, her leg in a cast, and us with a load of sleeping pills and pills to keep her leg from swelling in the cast. Too many pills.

Several hours later she had a stiff neck and her head began to tilt backwards. A friend, Laurence, and I took turns, pulling with all our might, our backs arched, to help her get her head forward again. Caroline laughed. We did too. It seemed like a stupid joke. But after a certain time no one thought it was funny. Suddenly I thought . . . tetanus . . .

I called the doctor. He spoke of "contractures" and discontinued the pills. Everything returned to normal.

Caroline spent her days reading and drawing. Laurence sped down the slopes.

When we got back, Laurence went to school all by herself. She was a little fretful. She said, "I'm fed up. Nothing ever happens to me."

Anne was delighted to have Caroline home. She loved her big sister. They had long games of *crapette* and Anne learned—it wasn't easy—to knit.

On April 23, I took the three girls to the Olympia to hear Antoine sing. At that time they called him "the king of the beatniks" or "the French Bob Dylan." Quite an exaggeration that was.

But the children thought him "super" and they were angry when we made fun of Antoine's *lucubrations.*

I asked for seats near the stage but on the aisle. Here, too, you never know: You have to be able to leave at a moment's notice!

When Antoine appeared, his hair flowing in long waves over his flowery shirt, there was pandemonium.

He undulated on the stage, the mike almost between his teeth. His band was excellent. Him I found pretty bad, no voice, no charm, no craziness. But the girls clapped like mad. Anne's hands were all red inside from clapping.

At the end of the show, a girl with platinum blond hair that streamed to her waist jumped onto the stage and began to dance. Applause. Whistles. Shouts. "She's Antoine's fiancée," one of the girls informed me.

Some fans, kept back by the police, tried to kiss the cuffs of Antoine's trousers.

My head felt like a pumpkin.

Afterwards I took them into the idol's dressing room.

The walls were plastered with drawings and photographs of naked breasts.

"I find them more fun than congratulation telegrams," Antoine said mopping his brow. "I want to have the craziest dressing room the Olympia ever had."

Then he came up with statements like: "I prefer making noise with amplifiers to making it with guns." Or, "I'm against the war and for the pill."

The last word went "tilt" in Anne's mind.

When we were leaving, she asked: "What pill'd he mean?"

"Singing pills," Caroline said.

"And for making hair grow," Laurence said.

It was a great afternoon.

The girls were growing up. Their personalties were developing. Each in her own way.

Caroline loved books—poetry in particular. Crocheting. Solitude. And drawing.

Laurence loved animals—horses in particular. Jazz. Company. And also drawing.

Anne loved tranquility. Silence. Cards. Everybody—and two persons in particular. And smearing paint.

Caroline devoured every book that fell into her hands. She had just read Boris Vian and was discovering Ionesco. Words enraptured her. Now and then you'd hear her laugh. When she was reading, nothing else counted.

Sometimes she declaimed passages to her sisters. If they seemed too distracted, she would shout:

"Come on! Are you listening or not?"

Then she would tromp back into her room, grumbling:

"You are *a*cultural, you poor . . ."

I had met Eugène Ionesco several times.

"What's he like? What's he talk about?" Caroline pressed me with questions.

When I told them a story, the three girls would climb on my bed, turning around like puppies before making themselves comfortable on a cushion, pulling at one another's sleeves, arguing over pillows, quarreling.

Words like "dumbbell," "dope," hurled back and forth. Often it came to "You simpleton," and "I pity you."

Finally they settled down.

I told them that Ionesco was a not very tall gentleman. He looked shy and he rolled and rumpled his hat between his hands when he entered a room.

"His eyes sparkle under his heavy eyelids and his nails are chewed to the nub."

"See," Caroline said, "they're the ones who chew their nails, intelligent people."

Anne smiled. Laurence shrugged her shoulders.

"He speaks in a low voice," I continued, "and says very funny things. Very slowly, one finger upraised, stressing each syllable, he tells his story: 'My Papa is Romanian. My Mama is French. I was conceived in France, but Papa said I had to be Romanian. So we all left for Bucharest where I was born.' "

"What's that mean, 'conceived'?" interrupted Anne.

"Don't ask silly questions," the two big ones said.

"Let her alone," I said. "It's when you begin a baby."

"I see," said Anne.

The two big ones giggled.

I resumed:

" '. . . It was fifty-two years ago,' said Ionesco, 'and if you stop to think that Methuselah lived to be nine hundred years old, he was just a kid at my age. . . . Then I came back to Paris. My Papa had a law doctorate, which enabled him to find a legal trick for leaving my Maman.' "

I also told them how once a number of us were in a restaurant with Ionesco. At dessert, he said:

"Who wants to share a cake with me? . . . I never eat more than a cake and a half."

Laughter from the girls.

Then I said that Ionesco liked to drink.

"Just like you!" the girls chorused.

". . . One day he went to Brazil by boat, and he was so happy to have time on his hands that he began to drink and saw absolutely nothing the whole trip. He doesn't even remember Gibraltar.

"He's always joking. When leaving, he said, 'Why don't we take off immediately for Hong Kong or Versailles, or for the suburbs?' The suburbs for him, that's Europe. Paris is a prison."

One other day I told them that the novelist, Le Clézio, who looks like a tennis champion and writes books incomprehensible even for most grown-ups, prefers to live his life at night.

"At night he works. He writes. Or takes walks through the old streets of Nice. He says that at night you meet strange people, fabulous characters, monsters. He told me that one very hot night he ran across an enormous buddha, an immensely fat man who inched along between two little boys waving big fans to give him some air."

Anne opened her eyes wide.

"And what does he do during the day, the fat monster?"

"He hides."

"Poor thing."

Caroline, who loved bizarre stories, said she'd like to see him.

And there was that other time when I took the three of them to see the shooting of *The Thief.* It took place first under the turn-of-the-century arcades of Rue Vivienne. Ten times they watched longingly as Belmondo, wearing a bowler hat and a wing collar, strolled under the arcade with Geneviève Bujold on his arm, she in a bustle, playing with a parasol.

"I've had it, Gen, right up to my chin," Belmondo joked on the sly.

"He's a genius," the three girls said.

Between scenes, he took refuge in a trailer where Ursula Andress was hidden. I went to speak with him there. The girls were mad that I wouldn't take them with me.

That same day we went to Joinville Cemetery.

There, Louis Malle was shooting a scene in which a man and a little boy wandered among the tombs. The little boy chewed his nails. The man scolded him and said, "If you like nails, chew somebody else's nails."

"That's funny," said Anne bursting into laughter.

"What, again?" said Caroline, referring to an article I had written recently about a starlet who never stopped chewing her nails. I had put that in my story and, in New York, where they're only too proud to display their good French, they made big headlines of: "Elle ronge *les ongles*"—"She chews people's fingernails."

One morning I took Anne and a little friend of hers to spend the weekend at Valgenceuse.

A mile from Senlis, the car coughed, hiccuped. Out of gas. On the autoroute, that's not so smart. I let the car coast to the shoulder and it stopped just behind another car in which a man was reading his paper.

I asked him if he could let me have a few drops of gas to get off the autoroute.

"You come at the right moment," he said, "if you could give me a franc and fifty for the toll, I could get off the autoroute too. I don't have a penny on me . . ."

"You see," Anne said to her friend, "when you're with Mother you never have to worry, there's nothing she can't solve."

Anne hated to hear me criticized. Another time, I ran out of gas on the autoroute. When I arrived home late, everyone called me careless, absent-minded, dumb. Anne said softly, "I love you."

Every night Zoulette wrote down in her diary a simple note about what had happened during the day. In the fifteen years that she stayed with us she wrote each evening a word or two about Anne, something like: "Anne is happy," or "Anne was operated on today." This little notebook served as a precious chronology for me. I would read one of these short notes and be flooded by memories.

Some things Zoulette put down in her notebook:

> *June 6:* Anne was nauseous at school. Her leg is much swollen.
> *June 10:* Anne, in full-dress uniform, went for lunch at Dupanloup. (school). Then on a pilgrimage to Montmartre. She was very tired when she came back and went right to bed.
> *June 26:* Anne is tired. Laura gives her a rose.
> *June 27:* Anne is eleven today. She is delighted with the suitcase her father gave her.

Anne spent the summer at La Chèze, hunting for mushrooms, going pedal boating, taking rides on the farmer's tractor, cracking beans, and picking currants. That's how the summer went by.

When we got back, the doctors put Anne on a new medicine—Imuran. She lost weight. She even returned to school.

But on October 28 Anne had terrible stomachaches and almost fainted on the bus. I took her to the doctor. That very evening she entered the clinic for an appendectomy. The same clinic, the same surgeon as for the biopsy.

He said it was none too soon. . . .

During the three days following the operation, Anne was in pain and vomited a lot. They administered intravenous feedings. She was weak.

On November 6, Régine gave a party at her nightspot, New Jimmy's, for some of her customers' children.

We thought Anne would be well enough to go. But we didn't figure on so much snow in Paris and on everything becoming more difficult and complicated. Crossing Boulevard Montparnasse and going to Régine's was suddenly such a perilous, icy, slippery expedition that I had to give up the idea of undertaking it with Anne. Even more, I was afraid that she'd be shoved around by the horde of mini-revelers who would have taken possession of the place.

Anne was very grieved.

Régine promised to come and visit her, her alone, one day. Which she did a few weeks later.

Anne was pretty proud.

The little children at the party—who now, grown up, come to Régine's alone at night—had quite an afternoon, dancing, popping balloons, fighting over comic books, and most of all, most of all, listening to their new idol, the pop star, Jacques Dutronc.

He snapped out words in rhythm that the kids howled back after him:

"ASPRO aspro . . ."

"LAVABO lavabo . . ."

"IMPRESARIO impresario . . ."

"PETIT PETIT PETIT . . ."

Anne used to wake me up every morning. When I was home. When I was not, she never went into my bedroom because it made her sad.

She would brusquely open the door and say:

"Get up, get up, come on! It's time! You're having lunch with me? You're having dinner here?"

"Zouzou. Leave me alone."

Then she would climb onto my bed. I yanked at her.

"Ouch . . . you're hurting me, ouch."

I always forgot she was sore.

We would kiss. And then quickly she would leave.

She would return to attend my bath.

Sometimes, when I fell back to sleep, she would say, "You're too much."

Sometimes too it was hard for me to surface. I would groan. Then she knew. She would go away, saying, "I'll come back when you're in a good mood."

When the telephone rang and I was not ready for it or I hadn't time to answer, I would say:

"Zouk, tell them I'm not here."

"Hello . . . hello? No, it's Anne"—people often confused us because of her low voice—"yes . . . no." She gets flustered—and I hear: "Mother says she's not here."

And then she would pull on her lip, as she used to do whenever she had a problem. . . .

"I didn't do it on purpose. . . . Oh well . . . they'll call again."

Often, when opening my door, she would announce, before saying hello:

"You know . . . I spat"—to spit is to vomit—"three times last night."

"You know . . . my leg hurts very much."

"You know, Michel d'Arcangues is coming for lunch."

"You know, yesterday I saw *La Grande Vadrouille* with Marc and Sophie."

"You know, my ear hurts."

Also she would tell me the news she heard on her transistor. It was she who told me about Walt Disney's death, about Bobby Kennedy's assassination. . . .

Anne adored General de Gaulle and prayed for him. When I went to his press conference, she said, "Say hello to him for me."

So, to tease her, I got serious:

"Yes, I'm going to raise my hand between two political questions and shout: 'General! Anne de Leusse salutes you.' "

"No, don't, Mother, you're crazy."

In February 1967, I took Caroline, Laurence, and Anne to spend a week at Klosters.

Anne was very thin and feeling well the beginning of that year. She got a great amount of good and, more than that, pleasure out of those eight days.

We were in a small apartment and Anne and I shared the same bed. What great joy.

Anne was bursting with activity. She was up first and prepared breakfast.

Then the moment would come for, "Mother, what should I wear?" Every morning the three girls asked the same question over and over again, and we piled up the tights, the socks, the bobbysocks, the underwear, and the overwear.

Then there were the shoes to lace and the skis to lug around.

We figured that a good three hours passed between reveille and the first run on the slopes.

Anne took some ski lessons, and she didn't do badly, I must say, not badly at all, on her skinny legs. She also went ice skating with Caroline.

I pulled her around on a sled or, squeezing her between my legs, raced down the hills on the sled. Anne screamed with joy and a bit with fear.

We deformed, murdered, the names of all the mountains. The Gotschna grat . . . the Brahmabubulle . . . Grôssetobel . . .

At night, we gorged ourselves with "Chesa" salad, to the sound of a rather old-fashioned band. We watched the Schweitzer-Deutsch couples, very formal and overdressed, taking their turns on the dance floor.

We went to bed late. It was a lot of fun.

"Health moves on . . . illness doesn't budge."

Every time we forgot about it, thinking it was asleep, the illness would rise up and manifest itself again.

No sooner would we take some liberty than it would, like an implacable jailer, call us to order.

It was always there. Crouched in a corner. Sly. Obsessive.

In March, the test results were very bad. Insufficient red blood cells. Too much albumin. Urea.

Anne suffered from headaches. Her blood pressure was high. She had a fever. She was nauseated. More and more often.

I took her to the doctor. He said she had a stomach ulcer. Not surprising, with all the medicines. But they gave her more: wafers to relieve the stomach pains.

In May the results of Anne's tests were even worse. Zoulette called the doctor who said he wanted to talk with me. Anne was nauseated and nauseated all next day. The following evening I called the doctor. He said there was nothing to be done.

That evening I cried.

Laurence came into my bedroom and I didn't hear her.

"Mother, what's the matter?"

"Nothing . . . Why?"

"You're crying."

"I was yawning."

"No. You're crying. Tell me what's the matter."

She planted her little black eyes on me.

"Tell me."

"You must be very nice with Anne."

"Why do you say that?"

"Just because . . . don't tease her too much."

"Why? . . . Is it serious?"

"Yes, it's serious."

"Is that what the doctor told you?"

"Yes."

Laurence turned away for a moment.

I look at her. She is beautiful. She looks like a colt, perched on her high legs.

She is intelligent. She works well. She is gifted. Everything is easy for her. But she is not very easy to take. Besides, no, everything is not easy for her. It's not easy to have a little sister who is ill.

I say, "Laurence, you must be more tolerant. And patient."

"I know, Mother. But it's not my fault. Anne gets on my nerves. She's always right. Zoulette is always on her side . . . you too, I might add."

She smiles a moment, and then that pout of hers.

"But you know why?"

"Yes, I know. But I love her, you know."

"I know. I understand."

She gives me a kiss.

"Don't worry."

No. I'll never show it again that I do. I must not show it. It isn't good for anyone. It doesn't help anything. People don't like people who let themselves go; what counts is to know that they're *capable* of letting themselves go.

Next morning, Anne came into my bed. I tried to fool around and laugh. But she only wanted to curl up and say nothing. She was totally listless.

She pressed herself against me. She put her cheek against mine and we remained this way a long time.

I called the office to say I wouldn't be in.

"You're sweet to stay with me," Anne said.

On June 3 I went with Kakoze to see Doctor Z.

That was the day when, gently, kindly, he told me there was no hope. That we should stop bothering Anne with all the treatments. That we should make her happy for the time she had left to live. Eighteen months. Two years perhaps.

Life toppled over in my head.

When I was back outside, I wondered how the sun could go on shining, the birds singing, the cars passing by, people walking, talking, laughing.

We had made plans to go to Greece for a cruise.

I had vaguely mentioned that maybe she would be able to come. But she kept talking about it every day.

I asked the doctor if Anne could go. He pondered. He hesitated:

"You know that the sun is very bad for her."

"I know. But she'll stay in the shade."

"The heat might make her uncomfortable," he said too.

"I know. But we'll find cool places. At sea it's never too hot."

"Swimming . . ." he went on in his soft voice. "That can be very dangerous."

"She won't swim," I said.

He smiled kindly, but his expression was one of sadness. Imperceptibly he shrugged his shoulders. After a pause, he said:

"Take her with you."

I thought it over for three days and three nights. Weighing. Imagining. Tergiversating. Searching. With my heart. With my head. Trying to understand. I was in agony. The choice was terrifying. How could I make a decision?

What part did my own adult selfishness play in this urge to give Anne some of the sweetness of life, while waiting to die? Waiting to die, which seemed to have been decided upon by men, but which, deep inside me, I didn't really believe in? Or in that hellish struggle to keep a hold on life at how much cost and suffering, how many tears and disappointments? What was the right thing to do?

To make her happy, or to make her live?

To stall for time by any means? Or let fate slip by? To survive, to live badly for as long as possible, or to die of pleasure?

What kind of an absurd, insane choice was that at eleven years of age?

To give up? Or to fight?

But she. What was best for her? Only she counted.

And it was quite evident that only life was important, even with its miseries. Misery is a part of life.

What nonsense. I was forgetting that Anne had far more wisdom and stamina than we.

We had to fight.

After three days of torpor, I woke up like a fury. It was urgent that something be done. To see other doctors. To act. Quickly.

I didn't want to hear about Professor Z anymore. I was mad at him. How stupid that was. (Afterwards I often thought of him. I heard that he often asked other doctors for news about Anne, that he never held a grudge against me, that he had understood perfectly. *He* was really good.)

I had his first assistant come to the house; Anne knew him well and liked him very much.

That was on June 6, 1967.

He told Zoulette (she wrote it down in her notebook but never told me) that "Anne couldn't last more than six months."

I asked him to work out an appointment with Professor X for me, the great kidney specialist, the head of the urology ward at Enfants Malades.

We went there on June 14.

He had a young face under his gray hair. He was bearish. His competence was recognized all over the world. He worked desperately hard. He was a fighter, a seeker.

It was obvious he didn't like emotional reactions. All that counted was the disease and the means to throttle it.

When I vaguely mention Greece, he raised his eyes skyward and said:

"Madness. Out of the question. You won't bring her back alive. Besides, I'm taking the child into my ward."

I shyly asked: "For a long time?"

"For as long as is needed."

He stood up, pressed my hand.

"Have the next one come in, please," he said to his assistant. That was on a Wednesday morning. Visiting day. In the large ward in Méry pavilion, many people, many children were waiting. There was no way to retreat. Inexorably, the hospital machinery had started to run. Now I would have to talk to Anne.

She was lying on her bed, when I got home, her eyes vacant, looking sad. Her legs and feet were very swollen. She had a headache.

I sat at the foot of her bed.

Two things I had to tell her: that she was not going to Greece, and that she had to go back to the hospital.

I looked at her. I hesitated. I didn't know how to do it. Where to begin? And once more she was the one to help me.

"Mother . . ." she said all of a sudden.

"What? . . ."

"I'm scared."

It's the first time she had said that.

"Why are you scared?" I asked lightly.

"I don't know. . . ." Her eyes grazed the mobile spinning on the ceiling. "I'm tired of being sick. I don't feel well."

"Listen, my Zouzou," I said then. "Don't you think we should wait a little bit before going to Greece . . . till it's not too hot? Till you feel strong enough to swim in the sun and eat everything you like in the tavernas? Don't you think that would be better?"

She listened. A tear rolled down her cheek.

"Maybe," she whispered. "But when shall we go to Greece?"

"When you feel well again. Soon."

"Yes, but when?"

"Listen, Zouk, I have another idea" (now I have to go to the end) "for things to go faster, we could go and see a doctor who has a very effective cure for the kind of disease you have; the only thing is that he never leaves the hospital; so . . ."

"No," she cut in bluntly.

"Nanou, listen. We won't stay long. It's worth a try. After that, you'll be able to eat anything you want, you'll become all thin again, we'll be able to do crazy things together."

"All right. If that's what you want."

That wounded me: "If that's what you want."

She was weary. She was sad. But I'm certain she was reassured too. At least I hoped so.

On Thursday the fifteenth, Zoulette left to spend the day in Arras, and Anne told her she was abandoning her. The seventeenth we stayed the whole day together, Caroline, Anne, and I. The eighteenth also, and I told her that she was to enter the hospital the next day.

June 19, I woke her up at eight-thirty. She was sad. But

she bravely got dressed. She couldn't swallow her breakfast.

Then I took her to Rue de Sèvres.

At the gate, I said that Anne couldn't walk, so that they'd let me go in with the car. "Of course I can walk, really!" Anne said, annoyed.

They let us go anyway.

We went up to the big building facing the central mall. On the pediment was written: INFANTILE GENETIC MEDICAL CLINIC.

We went up to the third floor, Netter ward.

The head nurse of the ward greeted us.

She was a tall, dark-haired woman, slim, energetic, and lively. We knew her.

"Good morning, Anne. Make yourself comfortable in number 18."

Number 18 is the fourth cubicle on the left.

Anne took off her clothes and put on her blue nightgown. She put her books in order on the radiator. Her games and her knitting inside the night table. Her alarm clock well in evidence on top of the night table.

She climbed onto her bed, pushed back the rough sheet because it was hot, and said, "I feel good."

From all around, they looked at us, kept watch on us. It's amusing, a new arrival.

The children who could walk gathered in a group in the passageway not far from Number 18. Two little girls ventured forward. One was a skinny little blond girl, the other, older, fat with dark hair. She wore little golden rings in her ears, a signet, and a necklace of glass beads. It wasn't long before we called her "The Queen of Sheba," I suppose because of her jewels.

"Good morning, good morning." They got acquainted.

"What have you got?" asked the little blond one, a finger in her mouth.

"I'm ill," Anne said.

"I had an operation," said the dark-haired one. "I'll soon be going on vacation to my big sister's at Les Sables d'Olonne."

"Oh, I see," Anne said politely.

"See that?" the Queen of Sheba went on. "That girl next to you, she's not allowed to drink. So, because she kept on drinking from the faucet, they removed the faucet."

We learned that there was a little blind boy, another who "walked" with his legs folded under him, a baby who cried all the time, another one who was completely tied down.

Anne listened, looked, smiled.

When I left, the dark one with jewels said, "Don't worry. I'll take care of her."

Anne winked at me. I left in a better mood. I knew that these little people were very well organized.

When I came back, there were three boys in Anne's room. One on the bed, one under it, and one pushing a little car along the walls and the bars of the bed. "Brrrrr. . . . Brrrrr. . . . Brrrrr. . . ." A racing car for sure.

The one seated cross-legged on the bed was buried in a copy of *Astérix among the Gauls.*

"This is François," Anne told me.

François raised the top of his nose. His eyes were bright and black. He went back to his reading.

I was hardly seated before the little guy under the bed grabbed my skirt and hoisted himself onto my lap.

"His name is Pascal. But he can't speak," Anne said.

Pascal adopted me. After a while I tried to have him get down. But he clutched at me. I kept him a long time, until a nurse came for him. "Just put him on the floor," she said.

I hesitated, and finally did. He then stole away at full clip, sliding on his bottom. Pascal could not walk either.

For weeks every time I came I saw his little head appear behind the door of the last cubicle at the end of the passageway and in seconds he'd be at my feet, stretching out his arms. I would bring him a toy or some candy. Pascal never had a visitor.

When I arrived the next day, Anne was dressing her Barbie doll, assisted by a blond little boy, very tidy and cute. Christian was his name. His mother brought him clean pajamas every day. He "lived" across from Anne.

"Zouk, are you feeling well?"

"Yes."

"Did you sleep well?"

"Yes."

"What did they do to you this morning?"

"Oh, blood tests."

She unfolded her arm, indifferent. I saw little red spots at the bend of her arm.

I looked at the metal frame hung at the bottom of the bed. A long list of test results was filled in. I read:

Blood iono
Urinary iono
Electrophoresis
Lipids cholesterol
N F S
VS

Thorax Knee Tibia Wrist X-rays
OT
EKG
Cell LE
E.E.G.
Erythrocytes
Leucocytes
Immunoelectrophoresis
Rh group
Antibodies anti-DNA
Immuno study
Hematocrit

"Mother, shall I be out for my birthday?" Anne asked.

"It's next week, you know, I don't think so. Maybe. I'll ask the doctor."

"But . . . I won't be able to have a birthday party here."

"Of course you will. You'll see. We'll invite everybody."

She brightened.

"You think they'll let us."

"You bet!" I said, jumping to my feet. "It will be a greeaat party!"

Anne laughed.

"Hush, Mother, you'll start a revolution."

"Exactly, Madame la Duchesse, and then they'll cut off our heads."

A tall black nurse passed by. She looked in at us, a little surprised.

"Hello, Anne, you having fun?"

"Yes," Anne says.

"She's a good girl," she said, "she never say nothing." And she went away dragging her feet. I heard her shout:

"Olivier! Olivier! Wait'll I get hold o'you!"

"Olivier is a nuisance," Anne explained. "He scrounges everything, he's never in his room, he drives everybody crazy and he runs so fast no one can catch him."

I learned that Olivier had been here for months and would remain for months to come. He was not really ill, but he had nobody to care for him. So they kept him at the hospital.

Olivier called Zoulette his "Granny."

Drop by drop the intravenous feedings continued. Each perfusion lasts six hours and Anne never flinched the whole time. She read and turned the pages with her free left hand.

For many days the tests, blood samples, X-rays went on.

Anne was on a very strict diet to decrease the rate of urea. No salt, no fats, no milk, very little to drink. All her food was weighed.

June 26, I talked to the intern on duty. I told him that tomorrow was Anne's birthday and I wanted to bring her a cake. But all cakes are forbidden, because how can you have a cake without butter, salt, or milk?

We racked our brains to find something.

"Lemon sherbet!"

"That's all right," he said.

June 27, Anne was twelve years old.

I came in the afternoon with a mountain of lemon sherbet. All the children able to walk came to have some and smear it all over themselves. The Queen of Sheba was there, the blond girl, the blind boy, the girl from 17, Christian, François, Pascal, Olivier, and all the others. We took some to the children who couldn't leave their beds.

The whole family had come, eight of us, all except

poor Laurence. You're not admitted under fifteen. So she made beautiful drawings of horses that Anne stuck on her window.

Anne received many gifts and all the children quarreled over them. We hastily stashed the Polaroid. And the big alarm clock I had brought too. This was a joke that the whole ward would enjoy for a long time. It was huge and red, it had a nose and round feet, wide eyes and a big smile. When you wound it up, it walked, batted its eyes, and rang like crazy.

Anne also received books, a lot of clothes for her Barbie, and a bound notebook that Nanny had brought. It was to write her memoirs in.

In the evening, Anne was exhausted but delighted. The nurses were not very happy. It's true we made a little too much noise. But, for this one time! After all it was Anne's big day.

When I had to leave, Anne suddenly became gloomy.

"Mother, I'd like to get into your bed."

She was curled up in hers, she looked like a very little girl, with big blue circles under her eyes.

"Don't forget to write your memoirs," I said as I left.

She nodded yes.

Later I found the blue book.

Here is what Anne had written in it:

Wednesday, June 28.

Today they took a blood sample. Also they made a urine test. They woke me up at five in the morning and asked me to stay flat on my back.

I made the alarm clock work for everybody, then I made the little two-and-a-half-year old girl eat.

Afterwards I went to the blind boy's room. Then I didn't feel well. So I went and lay down and it stopped. I lent the alarm clock to the girl who has the perfusions, and she found it very funny.

François and Pascal are playing in my room and I am writing my memoirs.

The doctors are passing by now.

The girl next to me does tapestry. Evelyne and the "Queen of Sheba" are in the room of the one who is sick. The boy across the aisle is coloring. I'll color too afterwards and read a story every night.

So long. Tomorrow I'll continue my memoirs.

Good-bye. Till tomorrow.

Anne

[with a beautiful flourish]

Thursday, June 29.

Today they woke me up at seven to put me flat on my back till ten. Then I took my temperature and weighed myself. I had breakfast. Afterwards we went hunting for cockroaches.

Anne

Friday, June 30.

Today I'm tired.

After breakfast I walked in the hallway to go and take a bath.

Today they removed my perfusions, that's why my arm hurts. I weighed myself. The doctor came to see me and he said that they'll resume my perfusions on Monday. Everybody is with me. We have fun. I dress my dolls. I put on new clothes on them.

I am writing the diary of my memoirs that was given me for my birthday which was last Tuesday.

I'm at the end of the Friday page. Tomorrow I'll continue my diary. Good-bye. So long.

Anne

[big flourish]

July first.

Today I had my temperature taken. Zoulette came to see me. Mother and Kakoze too. Mother won't come to see me tomorrow but she will come Monday the whole day. François and Pascal come every day to my room with Christian. The boy in 20 has a radio driven car. Christian is Nurse today.

Till tomorrow.

Anne

July 2.

Today they woke me up at 7:15, they took my temperature, they bandaged me and I washed myself. They took the perfusions off the girl in 17. She's combing her hair now.

Anne

Monday, July 3.

Today they woke me up at seven to take my temperature, then I went and bandaged myself, then I went back to bed after I washed my face and hands. Afterwards I had breakfast. Then the doctors came by, then I had lunch. Then Mother arrived with Yaya. Then Zoulette came to keep me company and Mother left but she'll be back. Now I stop my diary. I'll continue writing tomorrow. I say good-bye and so long. I'll continue my diary tomorrow. Once again good-bye and so long, signed

Anne

Tuesday, July 4.

Today they don't do a transfusion because they don't have the results but they'll do it tomorrow, so maybe I won't be able to write my diary.

Anne

Wednesday, July 5.

Today they woke me up at 6:15 for half my medicine, after that I went back to sleep. Then they woke me up around 7:25 or 7:30, after that I had my breakfast, I washed myself, then

I combed my hair and washed my hands. After that I told stories to the boy from 14, then I went back to bed to read and the doctors came by. I'm going to get my transfusion this afternoon but I won't sleep with it, tonight they'll certainly remove it. I'm stopping my diary because I can't continue, hugs and kisses everyone.

Anne

Thursday, July 6.

Today they woke me up at 6 to take my medicine, then I woke up at about 7 to take my temperature and weigh myself. Mother comes to see the doctor, they give me transfusions.

Anne

The little diary stopped here because Anne had no free hand left to write with.

Her two little arms were immobilized on splints. On either side of the bed, hung on metal uprights, were two bottles. The left one was full of a transparent liquid with all her medicines in it, plus calcium. The right one was full of blood.

Perfusion.

Transfusion.

Anne was very weak. Very calm. And it hurt me to see her the way she was. I started asking myself questions again.

At eight o'clock in the evening as I was leaving they removed the needle from Anne's left arm. The transfusion was over. But another full bottle was on the perfusion rack in order to continue the medications through the night.

The next morning, July 8, I found Anne with a swollen, discolored arm.

During the night the liquid had missed the vein and

flowed inside the arm. The morning nurse was the one to find it. But she hadn't yet notified the head nurse. I went to see her. She was visibly upset. She ordered compresses applied.

Anne said nothing, but she winced whenever her arm was touched.

I went to speak to the intern about it without telling Anne because she begged me not to say anything. The intern could do nothing about it. Nobody could do anything about it. Even in normal times there aren't nurses enough. But now it was the month of July, they were on vacation. The staff was reduced and you couldn't find replacements. And they're so badly paid, these hospital jobs.

It was at that time too that I talked about an artificial kidney with the Professor. He told me they didn't have enough of them, that they were forced to "unplug" the children during the night because they had no one sufficiently competent to watch over them, that he was waging a bitter fight with the administration to get more funds and staff.

I said, "If one day Anne can live only by means of a kidney machine, would she really be able to live?"

"We'll do anything to prevent that."

I knew it was not a life.

"But," he added, "there are many people, many children who live only thanks to them."

So I offered him, if not the total financing of a kidney machine, at least some help, some participation on my part.

He seemed moved, he shook my hand and thanked me.

And he never said a word about it again.

I thought of the waste.

I remembered something I heard, a little scrap of knowledge: Each bottle of mineral water or fruit juice sold for seventy centimes has a deposit of thirty-five centimes. Which means that the container and the contents cost the same amount.

For the hospitals in Paris alone, the bill for unreturned bottles comes up to 430,000 francs a year. . . .

Often, these first days in July, when I arrived, I found a big boy, Paul, seated near Anne's bed, reading to her.

He was gentle and shy. He blushed violently when I arrived. I must say that Anne did too, slightly.

He stood up right away and apologized.

"Stay with us," I used to say.

"No, no, I don't want to disturb you. I'll come back, if Anne wants me to, when she's alone."

"You know," Anne said, "he's at least sixteen. He's very, very nice to me. He often comes to ask if I need anything. He tells me stories and helps me do the games in *Pif Poche.*"

One day, going by his cubicle, I stopped in to say hello. He was reading Rousseau.

He was embarrassed to be caught lying down. He stammered apologies, blushed. He said he hoped to go soon to Bohemia.

I thanked him for being so nice with Anne.

"You know," he said, "she's marvelous. She's not like the others. I can talk to her. She's so full of wisdom; and so pretty too."

I could have kissed him.

One day, as I came a little late, I found Anne looking sad.

"Zouzou, I couldn't come any sooner."

"That's not it," she answered.

"You didn't have any visitors today?"

"That's not it," she said again.

"What is it, my love?"

"Paul left."

After a pause, she said:

"I told him I was leaving tomorrow."

"? ?"

"Yes, I told him that I was leaving too tomorrow."

She had put on that stubborn little face I like.

"Because he told me not to stay here too long."

At the end of July, a big envelope addressed to Anne arrived at the house. I took it to the hospital. In the envelope there was a giant postcard representing a sunset behind a big pinetree, on the seashore, and a little sailboat. Arcachon.

It was Paul.

Anne blushed with pleasure. She read, first silently to herself. Then aloud, slowly, with her gruff voice.

"First there is something printed, listen:

Serene and free as the air, not thinking at all
To dream lone and silent, perceiving the sea call.
André Chénier.

"Who is *he*?" Anne asks.

"A poet."

"Okay, listen:

" 'Hello Anne,

" 'I see that you had the good sense not to linger too long in the Netter ward . . .' "

Anne made a face, glanced at me, and went on:

" 'Trust the experience of an "old" man,' old is in

quotes," she stressed with a crooked smile, " 'don't haunt these holiday resorts except briefly and as seldom as possible.

" 'Forgive the delay; I finally got back from the Kingdom of Bohemia only yesterday. It's curious how hard it is, every time, to reaccustom yourself to the more or less peevish faces of our compatriots. You're really lucky to spend your vacation in that beautiful region of Corrèze.' "

Then he compared Arcachon's beaches to those of Dunkerque in 1940. Here I give Anne some explanations. And she goes on:

" 'All the same, don't eat too many currants. Leave some, if for nothing else than the preserves. Your stay at Netter must already be just a vague and distant memory.' "

Anne pulls at her mouth.

" 'But don't exhaust yourself and don't go too much in the sun; it's very funny giving good advice you don't follow yourself. It lends you some importance.

" 'I see that your mother' " (well, I say to myself, she wrote him) " 'is very understanding because I was really embarrassed and sorry to have talked so much nonsense.

" 'Kisses, Paul.'

"That's nice," she concluded.

I'm really moved to think of how kindly and good such boys are, boys like my nephew, Eric, who sometimes comes to spend the whole Sunday afternoon with Anne. He, a real tornado, stays for hours patiently playing checkers, *petits chevaux,* or *crapette* with her.

The sensitivity of a sick child—of anyone sick, I believe—is beyond belief; sickness makes them perceive more keenly their isolation and solitude.

Illness gives them so many reasons and occasions to

develop this sensitivity, which certainly makes them more vulnerable, but also wiser.

One must learn to patiently observe how sick children live in order to discover the treasures of kindness, tenderness, and wisdom that they possess and so often hide through modesty.

One could be tempted to take as a form of selfishness the fact that they seem to settle down in their own world, and that they sometimes fiercely defend its frontiers, but this is only their pattern of survival.

Anne was uneasy when we upset this pattern, either through negligence, or necessity, or because we thought it was salutary for her to unsettle her habits a little.

That's how the month of July rolled by. The hospital emptied, patients and attendants.

It was very hot. It was now possible to open the doors in the hallway and get some draft because there was less noise. Doctors were becoming scarce for the morning tour. We went cockroach hunting. I had distributed aerosol bombs, but we still found them slyly at home in the paper cutouts.

I brought watermelon. Anne loved it, but she was allowed only a small slice. We had no trouble finding customers to devour voraciously what was left.

Anne's cubicle was always full of children. She lent or gave away all her toys, all her books. She was gentle, generous, and understanding with them all.

Sometimes I lost my temper. When I saw that she was very tired, I wanted to chase the noisy horde away.

"No, it doesn't matter, let them stay," she used to say.

I let them. I loved them. She loved them too.

On July 25, I talked with Professor X. He said that Anne was doing a little better and that, everything considered, we could take her home, on condition that she not leave Paris, that she follow her diet rigorously and that we bring her every week during visiting hours.

Of course, I promised, I swore everything, everything, everything.

I returned to Number 18 to announce the good news.

"Swell!" Anne cried.

The morning of the twenty-eighth, Zoulette and I went to pick her up. She was ready. She had put on the little brown jumper I had bought at Ungaro's. She was a little thinner. She was very pale and delighted. We kissed Olivier, the last one remaining from the old guard, and we promised to come and see him very soon.

We spent two days and two nights, never apart. In the evening, Anne would lie on the drawing-room sofa and revel in watching television.

On July 31, I took her to the Hôpital des Enfants Malades. Professor X was about to go on vacation. He delegated his authority to a young blond doctor and entrusted Anne to him. We went to pay a visit to the little friends in "Netter."

On August 2, we went back again. It was something of a desert. With the advantage that we didn't have to wait for the blood sample the blond doctor has asked for.

Anne was very tired. She was nauseated and had diarrhea. She tried to hide all her miseries from us. She was so afraid of going back to the hospital. She was in a dark mood.

I left for La Chèze with Caroline to join Laurence there. I'd been neglecting them these days, "my poor two big ones," as Zoulette calls them.

At La Chèze, there was Tonton, the miniature dachshund Anne had received as a gift. Like Caroline he was born in May. He was the smallest "Taurus" anyone'd ever seen.

We sent pictures of him to Anne.

Every night we telephoned Anne.

Her voice was sad. On August 3, she said to Laurence:

"Régine has come to see me."

"Who?" Laurence shouted.

"Régine!"

"You lucky devil! She came alone?"

"No . . . yes."

"Yes or no?"

"With friends," Anne said with her calm, gruff voice, "but she left them on the landing."

On August 9, Anne had a high fever and couldn't move her leg.

On August 10 she was back at the hospital. Netter ward. Number 16.

Her father and her Grandma accompanied her that morning. When they come back in the evening, they found her in a cast. And under perfusion.

I suffocated with rage when I heard this.

"Was it so absolutely necessary?"

"The intern said it was preferable. He's afraid of osteomyelitis," said Charles, obviously upset.

"But do they have to have a cast up to the neck for a tibia?"

"I don't know. They didn't consult me. That's how I found her."

I went back to Paris.

Charles had had the cast loosened around the chest and under the arms. I could still see red traces. The sight revolted me.

I went to see the intern. I persuaded him to have the

cast opened on both sides. Which they did. Brutally. Hurting her: She admitted it to me afterwards.

Twice I arrived at half past one. I found her lunch cold on the night table. Nobody had come to make her eat.

"It doesn't matter, mother, I'm not hungry."

"All the same," I thought gnashing my teeth, "and what of the others? What happens to the others? The little ones who can't eat by themselves? The ones who can't move? Who have no visitors? Nobody to watch over them? To fight for them? To fill the gaps of indifference, of carelessness? All right, it's August. There are few attendants, and the few remaining are snowed under. It's vacation time! But what of those who have to stay, and spend the summer without sun, without tenderness, without a smile?"

And I'm going to Greece. I'm fleeing. With Caroline, Laurence, and Guy who calls Laurence "Princess Pistachio," and Mimi and Anne's buddy Michel. Just for a few days.

We told Anne we were going to the country . . . that we would be back in eight days. She asked no questions. She didn't want to know.

During my absence, Zoulette put down in her notebook that every day she read *Les Misérables* to her, that every evening her father came to see her, though he hated the hospitals. In mid-August she went home.

August 25: I remove the top of the cast and wash Anne with Mustela. Her father left early today on a trip.

August 26: I gave Anne a steak and noodles for lunch. Right after that she calls me. She throws up. She throws up several times.

> She has diarrhea all the time. I telephone the doctor. He's not there. I call the hospital. Nobody there anymore. I call Anne's Grandma. She comes. The telephone is out of order. So we call from the neighbors'. Finally we find a doctor from the hospital. He speaks of taking Anne back.

Every evening in Greece, in every island, in the post office of every harbor, I had a fight with the Greek telephone system. I watched for urgent telegrams that always take several days.

When I returned, I took Anne out of her awful plaster shell. "Come to me, my little snail." She hung on my neck.

With Zoulette's help, I plunged her in a bath. I put oil and perfume in it.

"How good it feels," she said. "Mmmmm, thank you, Mother."

Her skin was bruised and sore, her big toe red, swollen. It hurt.

Later we had to have the nail removed. It half-grew back, all crooked, and ugly. She found it atrocious. Every morning she observed it minutely.

"You think it'll look like it used to?" she'd say.

Then we didn't speak of it anymore. One little misery more or less. That lousy sickness that wreaked its damage right down to those pretty, slender feet!

August 31. Eric and Sophie arrived from Corrèze with Tonton. Tonton is very small, silken, cheerful. Anne was delighted.

The little dog jumped on her bed, licked her face, and disappeared under the sheets.

Anne squealed with joy.

Tonton thrust his muzzle forward, rolled on the rug, raced through the apartment, ears flopping, tail in the air (we call it his periscope). Then he raced back, slid, got into a crouch, once, twice, and somersaulted again and again.

"Alley oop! oop!" Anne said.

Oop! he was back on the bed.

To the very end, Tonton was to be Anne's inseparable little companion. Cheerful, faithful, loving. He slept in her bed.

But for months he made monkeys of us all, as Anne said. He would busy himself tirelessly emptying the shoe closet, hiding Anne's slippers, tearing up stockings, nipping at the curtains, eating the chairs, digging holes in the cushions.

And peepee everywhere.

We forgave everything. Once I had leaned a picture, not a Rembrandt to be sure but a pretty painting all the same, against the wall. Tonton chewed half the canvas.

At our house, we didn't attach too much importance to such things.

There were always a lot of animals in the apartment, most of the time brought in by Laurence. Back from school, she'd spend at least two hours feeding and caring for them. Then, if she had any time left, she'd do her homework.

There were four canaries that soon became fourteen. Three Bengali finches which in reality turned out to be nothing but sparrows (I had bought them at the bird market—one blue, one yellow, one green; in three days they had all turned gray), a turtle that died and dried up in the sun one summer. Fish. Ants, which Laurence observed in their glass habitat. A yellow cat that slipped away to the neighbors' by way of the balcony. A big hound that Charles had brought back from a distant island because it was bored there and that was supposed to be only a "transient" in the house. He stayed a year.

Anne was supposed to remain in her cast until September 25.

In reality she lay next to it. All day. It was so much too much for us, this instrument of torture, that I heaved it under the bed.

Anne was fantastic. She didn't move. "We won't tell anyone . . ." We were accomplices.

At night, out of caution, I put her back on the lower part of it which I had lined with cotton, gauze, and foam rubber.

We went regularly to the hospital for "checkups." And Anne would say, "Pack me up in my box." I wound her up like a mummy and when we got home I tossed it all away.

Finally summer ended. A sad summer.

Anne slowly regained her taste for living. It was a gift that she only seldom lost.

It was hard for her to walk. We had her go through rehabilitation exercises. She tired quickly. She had pains here and there. She was uneasy. She yearned for calm and silence.

Toward the end of October, Zoulette took her to Dupanloup, Anne's old school. The teachers and her classmates welcomed her enthusiastically. She came home very proud of herself.

But she was unable to go back to school.

I noticed she was becoming anxious. Concerning time. What time it was. She'd wind every watch in the house, every alarm clock. She called Time on the telephone to make sure we were right, and she asked ten times a day, "What time is it?"

One evening, she said, "Mother, what time do you have?"

"Eight o'clock," I said.

"You're crazy, it's a quarter to eight."

"But what difference does it make, Zouzou? What if I told you three in the morning?"

"I'd say you were crazy."

She laughed and threw herself into my arms. In her room she had hung calendars everywhere. Jumbo, the elephant calendar that her friend Stéphanie gave her for her birthday. And then all the calendars, from the postmen, the garbage men, the organizations for the blind. She wouldn't go to bed before she had, with her left hand, carefully crossed off on all her calendars the day that had gone by, or turned the little cardboard handles on Jumbo.

The evening of the last day of every month, the ceremony lasted longer.

Anxious over the organization of the house, especially when Zoulette wasn't there (which, thank God, was rare):

"Mother, who's going to take me to mass on Sunday?" she'd ask on Friday.

"Me, or Caroline, or Daddy."

"But what if Caroline is sleeping, or if Daddy isn't here, or if you have something to do?"

"But don't worry, there's always Carmen."

Or she said, "Mother, who will wake me up so I can start my homework at nine o'clock?"

At summer's end, she said:

"Mother, am I going to go anywhere this year?"

"Maybe not this year. But next year we'll go to Klosters, we'll go on a boat, we'll go to Greece, we'll go to La Chèze. We'll go everywhere."

"You think so?"

"I'm sure."

"But when?"

Our vagueness was insupportable.

She was anxious too, mainly over her illness. She was always on the lookout. She feared its attacks, its pernicious warnings. Every morning, she inspected the bottles lined up in a row on her small white wardrobe. When she saw that the level was too low, she'd come into my room and say:

"Mother, we're almost out of Cortancyl. I've only three wafers of Nepressol left. You'll have to buy some Reserpine" (or Antipressine or Tetracyne). "If you don't have the time, will you leave me the money?"

"But of course, Nanou. Don't worry."

But she would worry me to death. Sometimes I got impatient. I shook her. I sent her packing. And instantly I regretted it, as I saw her little mouth tighten, her forehead wrinkle in a frown, and her hand pull at her lip.

I'd say, "Lordy, get away from me," and if she left, crestfallen, melodramatic (yes, she liked to put on an act once in a while), I'd rush to her, lift her off her feet, and we'd waltz. She'd hug me then:

"I love you."

"I love you too."

"Whoopeeeee! Life is beautiful!"

For Christmas we all went to Valgenceuse. Anne insisted on going to midnight mass; but we were forced to leave before the Elevation. Anne was very tired. It really bothered her to be tired.

"Won't you be back for New Year's Eve?" she asked me.

"Hmm . . . no."

"You're sure you have to go?"

"Yes, no, not really."

"Then why go? I'm bored without you."

I went anyway.

Anne took long walks in the forest with Grandma, who also took her in her car to follow the hunt that Laurence and Nathalie joined on horseback.

She often stayed lying down and Zoulette read *The Odyssey* to her. They talked all the time about Ulysses.

It was 1968.

Anne had a hard time recovering from that terrible autumn. Among other things, her foot hurt.

We showed her to a bone specialist. When I told him the story of the cast, he shook his head in dismay. But of course he made no comment.

Almost every Wednesday morning we went to see the doctor at the hospital. Putting Anne into the ward again was often the question: The test results were bad; her blood pressure was very high. But everybody hesitated and went to great lengths to avoid it. It became an obsession for Zouk.

In March someone told me about a faith healer, marvelous I was told. Why not try, after all? What's the risk?

I told the doctor. He was skeptical, but intelligent and kind. He too said, "Why not?"

So I wrote a letter and attached as requested a lock of Anne's hair.

A few days later I received a piece of cotton and a bottle of water. You're supposed to take a mouthful of the water every morning and evening, and wear the cotton against the skin.

Anne did it all conscientiously. Of course, I told her not to expect a miracle. But she too never gave up hope.

Some time after that, the healer wrote to tell me to stop all the medicines. At that point I said no! I wasn't about to risk upsetting a balance, as precarious as it may be, that the doctors had tried so hard to establish. I mentioned it only to Zoulette, who said: "Oh, Madame, really! We have no right. It's too dangerous."

We continued with the cotton and the water . . . *and* the medicines.

In April, I spent a few days in a clinic for a minor operation. Anne often came to see me:

"Poor Mother," she said, very sorry, "she's sick."

"For once, it's me! It's my turn for a change, don't you think?"

"No, I don't want you to suffer! It's out of the question!"

When she said "It's out of the question," there was no point in arguing.

I could see how weary she was. As soon as she came into the room, she let herself fall into a chair.

I told her what things were like in the clinic.

"There is a night nurse, you know, who slept in my room and snored so loud she kept me from sleeping all night. And she was so sound asleep I dared not wake her, and besides she didn't hear me when I called her."

Anne smiled. She had had so much of this kind of life. . . .

The next day I didn't have a night nurse:

"Zouzou, you know what? I rang five times last night. Nothing doing. Nobody came. But one can manage on one's own, don't you think?"

"Oh yes, that's true."

I told her about a funny cleaning woman who distorted every word she uttered.

"This morning she slipped on some tulip 'pedals' and fell flat on her rear, then, when she was arranging a bouquet of roses, she said, 'They make a nice contrax with the others.' "

Anne broke out with one of her deep laughs.

Then I stayed home a few days.

"It's good the two of us quiet like this," she said, coming to settle herself in my room in the morning. "I'm not disturbing you?"

"No, baby mine, stay."

She worked a little. I helped her a little. But not too much.

"I have to work alone, or else the teacher will see there aren't any mistakes and she'll scold me."

"Oh no," I protested, "she'll think you're making progress."

This troubled her, so I didn't insist.

Afterwards, she curled up at the foot of the big bed and stayed there for hours without a word.

When friends came to see me, I watched her out of the corner of my eye. She'd listen for a while, then start to dream. She'd get lost in long reveries—the thread of them completely beyond me.

"Zouzou," I said abruptly sometimes, "what are you thinking about?" Or, "What do you think about this or that?"

"Nothing. I don't know."

Obviously I upset her. I wondered what was going on behind that broad, troubled brow. I wanted not to think about it too much.

That's when, for two mornings, Zoulette came to tell

me that she had the impression Anne was having trouble speaking when she woke up.

I said, "Oh no, you're imagining things."

"All right," said the poor Zoulette going off, looking insulted.

I refused to accept this new anxiety.

The third morning though—it was April 6—Zoulette rushed into my room:

"Madame, Madame, come quick, Anne can't talk."

It was that day, I think, that the most poignant episode in the tale of this filthy disease unfolded.

Nothing was spared her. Not even the sharpness of her lucidity.

Anne spent a week in the hospital. It disappeared as suddenly as it had come.

Then she came home for a week. For Easter. She watched the other children hunting eggs in the Valgenceuse park. But she didn't join them.

Zoulette noted: "She enjoys herself nowhere."

Anne was sad. She was afraid. Afraid "it" would come back.

Every morning, upon waking, she sat in her bed and proclaimed very distinctly, "Don't you see, Zouk, it's finished. Finished. It will never come back again, never, I swear."

I wanted to reassure her. I wanted her to recover her lightheartedness, her smile, her gaiety, her confidence.

She returned to Enfants Malades for a week, her diet even stricter, her medicines more numerous. But no matter: she was getting better.

It was at that time that the healer wrote me to resume medication!

One morning, Anne was in her bath and I heard her singing:

A horsey said to his mare
Marry me, marry me
A horsey said to his mare
Marry me and merry be . . .

And she went on:

The mummy said to the bear
Bury me, bury me
The mummy said to the bear
Bury me by the berry tree . . .

Through the door, I exclaimed:

"Zouk, you sing damn well!"

"You think so?"

I heard her laugh and: "You're making fun of me." She could be touchy.

"Not on your life! Who taught you that pretty song?"

"Caroline did, last night. She said it's not very smart." Fine. Clearly she's better.

Then occurred the "Events" of May—the riots of 1968. The girls were certainly interested in the demonstrations. A little uneasy too. I roamed around the Latin Quarter a lot, both for the paper and out of personal curiosity. I told them what I saw, especially the gags. "One, two, three four . . . we don't want your schools no more," was the slogan they liked most.

I came home "in tears," my eyes red and swollen. One night, on Boulevard Montparnasse, a tear-gas bomb burst at my feet. When I got home, my right calf looked like steak tartare. Anne was mad and forbade me to go "there" again.

But I did go back.

I told them how I had seen a lady in a white sailor suit

walking a miniature poodle through the halls of the Sorbonne (it was in the beginning, of course), while Cohn-Bendit harangued the crowds in the main Amphi; that some girls from good families took care of the babies of students who were busy hurling paving stones; that at the Beaux-Arts, where I had gone to pick up posters (and where I was told that I was only risking my life carrying them), I was surprised to run into several charming boys who had exchanged their starched collars for red scarves.

Because my job entitled me to ten liters of gas a day (obviously I couldn't use it all were I even to drive around all day), I syphoned the gas tank of my little Austin for my buddies and returned "to the line" time after time.

Anne found all this bizarre. I can't say she was wrong.

One morning we burst into fits of laughter.

I had broken a front tooth and the dentist had put in a temporary one to wait for "everything" to calm down. Actually, nothing was working then. All of France was on strike.

So. I had an important meeting; I was in a hurry; and there my tooth goes, plop, into the sink and down the drain. No wrench to undo the pipes, no plumber, no one available at S.O.S.* I was saved by the concierge who was fortunately on strike too and hiding out in his place.

And then there were actors enduring their flops at the Odéon, those who discussed the events of the day, drinks in hand at Castel's, cracking jokes.

"I just called a buddy at *France-Soir,*" said one, "I couldn't hear a thing, there was so much noise from all those coats turning."

*In Paris, an emergency repair service.

One afternoon, I picked up a student hitchhiking.

"So," I said, "you've just come from Charléty?"

"Oh no," he answered, "I'm not into that sort of thing anymore. I'm finished with being a student. I feel like doing something else now. To make my life's dream come true."

"And what could that be?" I asked.

"To be a model at Cardin's."

I gave him an introduction to Cardin's.

Another time, the day of a big demonstration against de Gaulle, I crossed Place de la Concorde, black with the crowds hurrying homeward, in this period of no public transportation, by foot. My eye caught a very fat woman who seemed exhausted from the anti-Gaullist demonstrations. I motioned her into my car.

"You're just coming from the demonstration?" I said by way of conversation.

She burst into sobs and whimpered:

"Yes, but [hiccup] we've lost General de Gaulle [hic], the poor man, what a pity to have this happen, [hic] let us pray for God to protect him."

The girls, and Anne in particular, were very worried about General de Gaulle and Pompidou. They were glued to their transistors or to the television, and the adjectives they called the others there was no arguing with.

The year 1969 was a beautiful one. The most beautiful, I think, in Anne's life.

In spite of the pain, in spite of the medication and the diet, in spite of the artificially induced plumpness, the fat cheeks, and cracked skin, in spite of the blood samples and regular tests, in spite of it all, she was happy.

There were no stays at the hospital.

We went to Klosters, Capri, Spetsai, Binic . . . And those are the only things I want to remember.

When we went skiing at Klosters, Caroline, Laurence, Anne and I, Mimi, Michel and Zoulette invaded the little dining room.

I handed the menu to Anne: "Order whatever you want."

"What about my diet?" she asked, puzzled.

"We can drop that for tonight. Tomorrow we'll see."

She was dressed all in red and she was red with pleasure. She ordered wiener schnitzel and fell asleep before dessert.

The next morning, the first ones up got on the phone to order breakfast. Anne began a collection of mini-jars of preserves.

Later we went to rent skis for "the big ones" and a sled for Anne. (We couldn't run the risk of letting Anne fall. Her bones were as fragile as glass, destroyed by the cortisone, something no one else yet knew.)

Every morning we rode up to the Madrisa in the little gondolas.

Anne came with her sled a little later to join us. She had the delicate job of reserving places for us for lunch around a large table on the terrace of that wooden kind of lodge that serves as a restaurant. The poor thing had a hard time warding off the fat ladies in tight ski pants who tried to put their authoritarian derrières into the chairs she was saving for us. On them she put her two mittens, her scarf, and sometimes her red cap with the pompom.

When we stopped skiing and arrived sweating and out of breath, we would sometimes find her freezing cold, or upset because little by little the feisty ladies had invaded the seats she'd been saving.

So I would take her in my arms and slide down the slope on her sled, until her face would glow again.

On February 18, Michel was thirteen years old.

We had a big dinner at La Chesa, *the* place in Klosters. Anne presided with Michel. At the end of the dinner, the band gathered around the table to squeak out Happy Birthday on their violins. Michel was so embarrassed we thought he would vanish under the table. Anne said, "Poor boy! Can't you see you're bothering him?"

Laurence asked Michel:

"Do you know the plural of *petit beurre?*"

"No, what?"

"*Des touyoux.* Because" (she sang) "*Un p'tit beurre, des touyoux . . .*"*

Michel and Anne strangled themselves laughing.

Another joke they were crazy about:

"Mr. Douyou is sitting on a cactus in the desert. An Englishman comes up to him and says: 'Do you speak English?' *Non, Douyou s'pique le cul.*"**

We all drank champagne, and we were as stiff as pokers.

On our way home, we even made a short stop at a nightclub. Anne and Michel were scandalized because there was a hen tied up in a corner with the job of laying an egg a day.

"That's what nightclubs are?" the two of them said, disappointed.

"It's too noisy here," Anne said, "I'd like to go home."

*The joke is that "*Un p'tit beurre, des touyoux*" sounds in French like the English "Happy Birthday to you." Laurence's riddle is nonsense, and its answer, "*des touyoux,*" is a grammatical coinage for the purpose of the pun.

**For the purpose of this joke, a Frenchman's name is Mr. Douyou. To the French ear "Do you speak . . ." sounds like "Douyou s'pique . . ." which means Douyou pricks himself: M. Douyou, sitting on a cactus, is pricking his ass.

We slipped and slid our way home. Zoulette was all the time losing the anti-slipping hooks she had tied to her fragile boots, so she could hardly remain on her feet while we scratched around in the snow looking for her hooks.

On other nights, the children went bowling, or played cards, squatting on their heels in their room.

Until, finally, it was time to leave.

During all those years I'd worked on Rue Cambon (the paper was only four doors from Chanel) and parked my little car there, I had accumulated an impressive number of tickets. There were so many "butterflies" in my car that one of the guys from Austin said he could paper his garage with them. There were more at home too. Every morning, with the mail, the concierge brought a little pack of yellow, blue, or pink parking tickets. They changed the color periodically.

I had given up paying, hoping for an amnesty that would bring me up to date.

Sometimes a man, very friendly I must say, rang the bell at seven in the morning so he'd find someone home. He was in charge of collecting money from the diehards.

Sometimes I paid; more often I said, "I have no money." And the man would leave, apologizing.

This worried Anne:

"Mother, what if they take you to jail?"

"You can come and visit me, bring me pretzels, and then at last I'll be able to rest."

"But I don't want you to go to jail. Mother, you're too much."

I also received large blue-gray sheets covered in an indescribable jargon that went on about seizure, imprisonment for debts, etc. I was almost a threat against national security!

Toward the end of March, one morning, I received a phone call from Anne at the office. She was in a panic:

"Mother, there are two gentlemen here. They say they've come to take the furniture."

"What for?"

"They are process servers. It's because of the tickets! I told you so!"

"Okay, so listen carefully, Nanou," I said. "Tell them to take the benches in the vestibule, the red chairs, the table in my room, and the green sofa."

"But, Mother . . ." She was appalled. "What's Daddy going to say? You're crazy."

"Listen to me. Listen carefully. Be sure to tell them to leave the metal coffee table in the drawing room, the Colombo, and the leather bags. Go on now." These were all the things I liked.

I waited.

"Hello, Mother, listen, they say they can't choose. Besides, they say they'll be back. They're making a list now."

"Good. See you later, Madame Zouk. Don't-worry-about-a-thing."

Some time later there was an amnesty and we didn't see the process servers anymore.

During April, I took Anne to spend four days in Corrèze. As we drove in the car we played "if he or she were . . ." We took turns picking the name of somebody well known, whom the other tried to guess with questions like: "If he were a flower, what kind would he be?" If he were a house? a car? An animal? A country? etc.

On both the trip down and back we stopped at the

Motel de Sologne where Anne perched on a stool and ate a hamburger at the counter.

In April we went to see the Bauhaus exhibition, which thrilled Caroline.

Anne went with Zoulette to see *L'Auvergnat et l'Autobus.*

On the twenty-fourth, I bought her two dresses, one terrycloth and the other pink-and-white linen in a mod pattern.

On the twenty-seventh Anne went with me to vote.

Anne played the piano, walked Tonton, slaved over her arithmetic, built another mobile, went with Yaya and Juliette to the Jardin d'Acclimatation, was busy being helpful around the house, read a lot, played cards and won every time.

I went to see the rehearsals of *Hair* at the Porte-Saint-Martin; I had promised to take Anne, but I only told her about it.

In May we took a four-day boat ride in Italy. Even better, my friend Bombom came with us, and Anne adored Bombom, her extravagances, her wit, her accent, her manias, her hats, her affability, her maladies. No one could make Anne laugh as she could.

We took a little plane to Naples. Anne signed the flight log with a grand flourish.

In Naples, we boarded the boat and Anne settled herself in a cabin facing mine. She put her things in order. She was very neat. The only one in the family who was, by the way. She was so happy that she threw herself into my arms every five minutes to prove her joy and gratitude.

"Thank you, Mother, oh! thank you Mother!"

In Amalfi we went bicycling on the harbor. We ate a pizza in a bistro and a lot of fresh mozzarella aboard the

Madreperla, which we called Mère des Perles, Perle des Mers, Merle des Pères, etc.

We visited Positano, Conqua, and the Esmeralda grotto. Anne was fascinated. The Italian who rowed us about inside this high grotto aimed his pointer at the ceiling with its strange, tormented rocks, announcing "Napoleone!" and "Garibaldi!"—or under the water to show us the bones of a giant fish, a knife, or, in one place, a rock formation like a creche.

To Anne, it didn't matter a bit whether they were natural or not.

"Look at the ox, the wise men, and the sheep, over there!"

Then we went to Capri.

We circled the island. We swam in an inlet behind the lighthouse. Not Zouk, though, the water was too cold, and—well, enough is enough. She was careful to protect herself from the sun under a big straw hat. She had also a parasol which she steered in the right direction to protect her feet and arms.

It was nearly perfect.

She was wearing a water-green terrycloth sailor blouse, the color of her eyes, and white linen slacks. Of course the zipper kept pulling open over her badly swollen middle, and from time to time, when no one was looking, she'd check the zipper, but she had nearly forgotten "her misfortunes," as Zoulette called the disease.

In the evening we strolled hand in hand, window-shopping in the narrow little streets of Capri. We had left the others for a moment to their Camparis on the terrace of the Hotel Quisiana, so we could go and buy gifts for Zoulette and Grandma. Anne chose a little coral heart for Zoulette.

Then we went to have dinner at La Campannina where the guitarist warbled his Neapolitan songs and made eyes at Anne. She was in heaven and got it all down on her tape-recorder.

We gave her a little enamel bracelet from Chantecler's, which she didn't dare put on for fear of breaking it, she liked it so much.

When we got back to Paris, Anne went around in a daze and there were tears in her eyes.

Zoulette wrote in her notebook, "Anne cries for Italy."

And almost immediately we left for Greece.

Professor X had given the green light, with an introduction to and the address of a pediatrician in Athens.

And off we went. The same crew as at Klosters, plus some others.

In Spetsai Anne collapsed on her bed and said: "At last. I'm here."

"Listen."

We could hear the hooves of the horses and the little bells of the fiacres. Cocks answered one another in the night.

"Smell."

The scent of jasmine filled the air.

"I feel good," she said.

We stayed there three weeks.

Every morning, Anne had fresh yogurt that a woman all in black brought in large flat baskets. Then we went down the steep road to the harbor. Laurence picked up figleaves for an old goat that bounded from the back of a thorny garden as soon as it heard us coming. A little farther down, we watched a column of ants at work one day, crossing the road.

At the harbor, Panayotis waited for us in his old tub, his fat belly bulging out over his pants.

Chug . . . chug . . . all the way to the Peloponnesus, across from the island, where there was a soft, sandy beach. Zoulette and Anne had found a little corner of shade in the hollow of a rock under a pine.

While we fooled around in the water, Panayotis slept, stretched out on the extreme edge of his boat. We wondered how he managed not to roll overboard.

Anne was allowed to swim for short periods in the warm water. She grumbled when I made her get out. And she returned to her rock shelter.

I watched this weighed-down little figure, with its uncertain gait, going off, and I turned away.

I repressed the bitterness and anxiety. I thought of the courage she had to have in order to be happy. It was her greatest virtue.

When the coolness of the evening came, we'd go for a walk on the *dapia,* the harbor square where everyone congregated and everything happened.

Anne munched pistachios—just a few on account of the salt. One day I gave her a taste of ouzo.

"That's nothing," she said; "it's just like paregoric."

In the evening, almost every evening, we went down to Vassili's, the tavern on the harbor. We pushed the tables together so we could be together and not to be in the way of the fiacres. Each of us went and filled our plates, digging into the huge copper pots that bubbled on the stoves. It smelled of oil and thyme. Anne liked the meatballs especially.

Zoulette got used to retsina. She tried to learn a few words in Greek, and then gave it up. Reg had told her she should answer "Maria Callas" or "Kon-Tiki" to everything, which she ended up doing and which gave Anne a good laugh.

Caroline had "her gang," and we hardly ever saw her. It griped Laurence not to be part of it.

But on the evening of her fifteenth birthday, Laurence made up for everything: she danced all night.

Anne was all gloom because we sent her to bed before going to the nightclub; she said, "Next year it will be my turn. I'll go dancing all night and go out with boys."

One night, we really had a ball in Hydra and we came home at sunrise. The light was soft, the sea was flat; but Zouk saw nothing of the return trip, she was sound asleep, rolled up inside a blanket.

She loved to watch the Déon children playing around. They went through life totally naked and looked like little Indians. Except that little Alexandre would modestly go apart when he put on his pants; Anne thought this was cute but not so surprising. Curiously, children have a natural sense, a good taste, in their manners. It's really less immodest to be naked than to take off or put on one's pants. When one is three one knows this very well.

Anne also liked the big modern house near the place where we went swimming among the rocks. At night, its huge roof terrace was strewn with children who had dragged their mattresses up there to sleep.

July 20, and we had to leave! I, because I had work to do, Anne because she was having frequent abdominal pains and because "one mustn't overdo."

In frightful heat heightened by the ceaseless shrilling of the cicadas, We took a fiacre to the top of the hill where the helicopter landed.

Flying over the lighthouse peninsula we saw them all,

our friends, waving good-bye to us. We were both sad, but each of us—so as not to upset the others—pretended not to care.

"It's not because of me you're going back, is it, Mother?" Anne asked.

"Not at all. I have to work. And also I didn't want to go back alone; that's why I'm taking you with me. To keep me company."

"But you're not sorry?"

"Of course not. It was plenty for me. How about you?"

She wasn't really convinced.

"Will we come back next year?" she asked.

I answered, "Sure. And we'll stay the whole summer."

We had a distant glimpse of the Acropolis through the mist.

I said, "You know, it's just as beautiful from far away."

She was pressing her head against the window.

I added, "The heat is overwhelming up there and you have to climb a long way."

"All right then," she closed the subject, "we'll do it next year."

I remember that we went to the restaurant across from the airport, because we still had a lot of time before the plane took off. I remember that Anne put one arm around my waist and that she took long strides to keep in step with me.

She radiated:

"Mother, I love being alone with you. Let's make the most of it."

We chose a table for two under a bower. We decided to forget the diet and Anne ordered melon, salad with feta cheese, and ice cream. We really enjoyed our last Greek lunch, just the two of us.

On the way through customs Zoulette joined us. She had bravely taken the boat the day before to tour Athens, and she'd seen everything. She was worn out, but the only sign of her exhilarated exhaustion was that her hat was slightly off-kilter. We bought pistachios and leather strings with blue glass eyes attached.

The 707 was almost empty; we each occupied three seats home.

The doctor came the next day and found Anne "in great shape." And she left right away with Zoulette for Corrèze. Her disease had once again disappeared momentarily, though we knew it would be back.

I had given her a light blue Cadie motorbike for her birthday and she spent her time going putt-putt over the roads, forgetting her aches and pains, her regrets, her sorrows, and even her loneliness when Zoulette went on vacation; forgetting everything on her precious Cadie. Now at last she could keep up with the gang of cousins and farmers' kids. With her Cadie, she was part of the gang. She kept to the right and the toughest of them kindly led the way. I rejoined her only at the end of August and watched her going back and forth between the bakehouse and the farm, her helmet strapped onto her head, her blond pony tail waving over her straight back.

On my way I had stopped at the Lalannes and told Anne that Claude was making new jewels which were molds of lips and navels, fingers and even "bozooms."

"But who would let her bozooms be molded?" Anne asked me, intrigued, a little shocked.

I told her that they were of a very nice metal and that they were jewels to dress up in, and some day people wouldn't want to put on anything else.

She answered back right to the point that it wouldn't be very soft or very supple either, and she asked:

"Maybe Mme Lalanne could make me a nice nail for my big toe?"

"Certainly she can."

And I promptly forgot all about it.

August 21, we took Tonton to Vicq, where he was born, to be married.

There were a lot of little female Dachshunds there, identical to Tonton. He didn't know where to begin and we hardly recognized him in the middle of this harem. All the little dogs raced after one another, round and round in front of the house. Suddenly exasperated, Tonton got frightened and fled inside to find shelter under the furniture.

In the end, we left him there two days, and Anne was very worried about him the whole time. And he got married. And he had children like himself, rich brown like mushrooms.

Zoulette invited Anne to Binic. She left September 5. She was bored there, but she never said so openly. Zoulette sensed it though, and I could guess as much from her letters. All the children were gone and the weather wasn't good enough for going to the beach. To top it all, poor Zoulette couldn't find a television to rent. No serials, no Shaddocks, no Daktari. So it was simply decided that she would come home by the next train. She told me the news gently but firmly on the telephone.

That very evening, however, there was a strike and no trains.

It was a big disappointment. Anne was tormented by the idea that Zoulette would take umbrage or be sad at her inexplicable hurry to get home. And indeed she was. Zoulette tried in vain to get her a lift and Anne finally took the first train on September 18.

"I missed you, I wanted to see you," is all she said getting off the packed train.

The last three months of that year went by quietly. No surprises. No attacks, no shocks; the disease seemed numb, as it often was in winter.

Zoulette helped Anne to do her homework, and listened to her recite her lessons; she gave her her spelling dictation everyday. She had her repeat: "When there are flats in the signature, you're in the key of the next to the last flat"; and Anne would play *Vivo e giocoso,* a gigue, a sonatina by Clementi, or an écossaise by Hummel. There were also *Les Exercices de Mlle Didi* (the name amused her).

I taught her some English words. She got twisted repeating them and she'd sputter with laughter, and usually forget them by the next morning. But so what.

Every afternoon she'd walk Tonton and a big companion dog with melancholy eyes and a very long nose who ran like a thoroughbred horse. Falco pulled Anne on his leash and dragged her on mad races that she had trouble keeping up with.

In November I had to leave for South America. We spent every minute of the day together. Anne was all melancholy and tender as she was every time I had to leave, and, as every time, vague feelings of guilt invaded me. Resolutely, I repressed them.

She said nothing, she did nothing to keep me back, but I read a thousand prayers in her eyes, which I pretended not to perceive.

Sometimes she rolled herself into a ball in my suitcases, like Tonton, and refused to get out until I put my foot down. Then she'd say:

"Oh please! I was only joking."

To tell the truth, I never really put my foot down with her.

The day after my departure, Zoulette put in her notebook: "Anne cries for her mother."

For the three girls I brought back necklaces made of crystal fruit and many-colored glass beads that I had bought at the humid airport in Dakar, ponchos from Argentina and *figas* from Rio.

I was still sunburned and when Anne wrapped herself around me our contrasting colors made me see all the more the pallor, the transparency even, of her skin and the blue of the blood vessels so visible under it.

My stories about immense beaches dotted with coconut palms, of unbelievably colorful sunsets, which, like a curtain being drawn, turn the day into night in an instant, of monkeys who snatch your cigarette to delicately burn off their fleas, of huge butterflies, marvelous birds, Pelé's thousandth goal and the pandemonium at Maracana, macumbas on the ocean front—everything I told them, till late into the night of the day I returned, was interrupted by:

"You lucky!"

"What about us? When are we going?"

"When do we leave?"

"Oh! Uh?"

Or even: "It's disgusting! you're too lucky."

At the end of the year, Anne carefully sorted out the toys, books, games, and clothes that she wanted to give to the young children at the hospital or for the Christmas party at Dupanloup. She gave her little piano to Juliette and her sewing machine to another little girl.

She gave everything away, except of course for what related to very special memories, such as the big red alarm clock with the long seductive eyelashes. She never tore up a letter or a postcard. They were in order in a cardboard box that she herself had made at school, and her most recent mail was clipped together with a long metal feather. All of it put on the shelf at the head of her bed.

Just before Christmas, she went out alone, all mysteriousness, in the afternoon "to go shopping."

When she got back with little packages under her arms, she had a sad and worried look.

"What's the matter, Nanou?"

"Nothing," she said and she went into her room and closed the door.

Her sisters drove her crazy with: "Show us! What's in the packages? Stop hiding things! What did you buy us?"

And then: "You're richer than we are! We're sure that you hide your money in a sock."

Anne shrugged her shoulders; she was obviously put out and there was something on her mind. Poor thing! Finally she opened her wallet, turned it upside down. It was totally empty. With tears in her eyes she said:

"All my money's gone . . . and I haven't finished my shopping."

The tragedy was remedied.

The day after Christmas, the "two big ones" left for the mountains to ski for a few days. It was impossible to send Anne, and she cried for her sisters.

I canceled everything, therefore, and decided to spend New Year's Eve with her. We went to the Carters' with Kakoze for New Year's dinner. Laura and Anne sat, just the two of them, at a little table at the end of the big one, and they gorged themselves with caviar.

Anne and I got back to Valgenceuse before midnight,

but we waited and wished each other Happy New Year at least fifty times before falling asleep, kissing each other like crazy.

"Happy New Year, my darling little Mother!"

"Happy New Year, beloved Zouk!"

Happy New Year!

IV

IT WAS 1970.

"Madame Zouk,

"It was fun on January first when we stayed upstairs the two of us hidden in my room, curled up in my bed. There were lots of people downstairs and the blurred hubbub of conversation came up to us in snatches by the main stairway.

"You were reading one of your books from the *Fifteen Stories* series and it seems to me I was reading a book in English, but lazy as I am, I stopped to read one or two short stories with you. Kakoze brought sandwiches and petits fours up to us on the sly. We felt good. Quiet. We had promised to come downstairs later. But when we finally did come down, no one was there.

"Toward the end of the month you had an inkling that Zoulette might possibly decide to work in May for some other people. You were furious, poor Nanou. First you said, 'Out of the question!' That was Act I: no compromise. Then, after some reflection, you thought it was not right to tyrannize Zoulette, that her absence wouldn't be for that long, that she'd worry if she saw you sad, and that she'd come often to see you.

"So you said, 'Okay, go if you like. But you're not going to tell the other little girls all the things you tell me.'

"That was Act II; acceptance; you resigned yourself but with a few restrictions.

"Act III always proved that you were perfectly capable of managing for yourself, right? You even gave proof of a surprising autonomy.

"I know you weren't happy alone, but listen: you were never really alone. The only thing was that for you solitude began with the absence of one or the other of your 'guardian angels,' as you sometimes called us, Zoulette and me.

"Then too, you were not one to be led, when neither of us happened to be around. You couldn't stand an order coming from elsewhere; you even said that nobody except me, Zoulette, and Daddy 'had the right to command you'!

"You had it all pretty well organized though. In the margin of your tablet I saw, one day, that you had written: 'We'll have to ask Daddy or Mother if, yes or no, they're going to take us to school tomorrow morning.'

"We were real bores never knowing what we were going to do: you had to ask the same question ten times to get an answer.

"You were stubborn sometimes, and you asked questions with a patience that nothing could put down. While *we,* we would talk about something else, change the subject, even whistle (which was rude, I grant you); and you, you would take it easy, even showing a polite interest in our lucubrations; then 'yes, but' and you would repeat the question again.

"You didn't like so much being teased, poor Zouzou,

sometimes you even got mad and bluntly said 'oh shit' to your sisters when they were teasing you.

"When Daddy called you in a long-drawn-out voice: 'Zouououk!'

" 'Yes.'

" 'Zouououk!'

" 'What?'

" 'Come, I have something to tell you.' And he'd say the same thing over and over again in even longer-drawn-out head tones:

" 'You're driving me craaaaazy!'

"Then you quietly shrugged your shoulders.

"Once in a while Peaceful Caroline had bursts of joy accompanied by verbal delirium. One day she had made a sketch of the two of us embracing on the drawing-room sofa. It was impossible to make out whose arms and whose legs were which; at the bottom she had written: 'Mother has a big darrière but Anne's is three times more important if one considers the volume occupying a distinct place in her anatomy.' At that you called her an idiot. And there was more: 'Mother also has feet of a considerable length which call for one to dwell on them before pursuing this rather particular overall description. In fact those feet offer the particularity of moving through an order from an umbilical influx itself set in motion by a winch coming from the left lobe of the cervical iris. Another observation: those feet totally refuse to do their job when the upper part of my mother is slightly under the influence of alcohol.'

"You turned your finger round and round at your temple, raised your eyes skyward, gave me a kiss and said, 'Poor Mother, I pity you having such a daughter.'

"Caroline and Laurence were out of breath from laughing.

"In February, I went to the Elysée for an article about the Pompidous before their departure for America. I remember that you and Zoulette accompanied me to the entrance. There, too, I said I would take you, some other time . . .

"Afterwards I told you that Mme Pompidou had shown me every part of their private apartment: their room with the Odilon Redons (remember how mad I was when they printed Odile Rodin in the paper? Do you? True, it didn't mean much to you). The 'weird' bathroom, as Mme Pompidou calls it, like a carousel, with the bathtub buried among evergreens, a dressing table and a washstand around a central shower which is a big pipe in smoked glass. I don't think you thought it much of a 'palace,' in your terms, as in *The Thousand and One Nights* for instance. And, after we had crossed a long, red corridor, with many paintings by Hartung hung on the walls between numerous doors, Mme Pompidou said wittily: 'Before we came, it was like a hallway in the Hotel Victoria in Aix-les-Bains; only the shoes outside the doors were missing.'

"I had also been shown the pictures of the grandson and learned that he had two teeth at three months.

"At that point, you, like a connoisseur, made a moue of admiration.

"Zouzou, forgive me for having stayed so long in Brazil. You were very upset, very sad, every time I sent those telegrams, especially the one that arrived after the plane I was supposed to take. It was not planned, I swear; it happened just like that, pftt, a few minutes before leaving; once, even, we were almost at the airport and someone said, '*Vamos a Buzios*' and since we are a little crazy—as you know—we failed to turn right and went to Buzios. But as there is no telephone, no electricity, in this little harbor, just little black pigs in the main street, it was hard for me to let you know. You didn't believe me, did you?

"I thought often, all the time, of you, you know, though it might not have looked that way.

"I remember that one day we arrived on an immense, deserted beach in Bahia, and I found a ring, the loveliest ring I'd ever seen. It was in wood with a red glass bead inlaid in it. I hesitated before taking it, thinking that perhaps it was a gift for Yamanja, the goddess of the sea, then I picked it up anyway in the white sand; later on an Indian woman told me that it was a token of very good luck and happiness, so I kept it with me all the time. You know that it's broken now.

"On that beach I loved to watch a little black boy trotting on his donkey, squeezed between two huge, round baskets. He came to us, brandishing a machete almost as big as he was; from a basket he took a coconut and halved it in one stroke. We were afraid the knife would slip down to his bony little knees. But it didn't. And we drank that tasteless juice which seemed deliciously cool. Then the little rider went on his way, stopping here and there in the shade of a cluster of coconut trees.

"You would have liked that scenery so much; I would have so liked to take you there some day. But, as you know, there's too much sun in that country for you.

"When I came back, it was Caroline's birthday. I took you to Castel's before dinner and Jean bought a round of drinks. As for you, you drank water. You looked around you everywhere. You were not happy that I took you home. I gave you your dinner on the corner of a table; we were just the two of us and, you know, I deep down wonder why I didn't let you have dinner there too; in the name of what, in the name of what convention? Please forgive me because I know that you cried all night in your bed. You were unhappy, staying home all alone.

"I agree, those Rembrandt drawings we went to see one Sunday were a little austere, but you did admire them (that was the period we decided to do 'intelligent things'). All the same, you found the Egyptian galleries and the sarcophagi more fun, let's say more entertaining.

"You remember that when we left, there was a guy who went after us to sell us stupid books for the benefit of I don't know what, and I tried to refuse, but you said we should buy some, 'to be nice to him.' I was annoyed because he was really insisting too much, he was too much of a leech. Finally I gave in.

"Now I always buy books that are sold in the street. I don't even argue. And I don't even look at the titles.

"Another Sunday, we went to the Flea Market. There were six of us at least strolling about single file among the displays of everything and nothing. We found T-shirts ('petits cheurts' as you said) for ten francs, the kind with spots all over on purpose; you were crazy about them at that time. Caroline chose a mauve one, Laurence an orange and you a blue. Your favorite color. Afterwards I remember that Fred took you for a little ride on his motorcycle. I can still see you, clutching him, a radiant and proud look on your face, vanishing at the corner of the street. Then you said, 'We'll do it again soon, won't we?' 'Me too, me too?' said Laurence. You were elated.

"It was fun to take everybody's blood pressure. It bothered me to have to squeeze your little arm every morning and every evening in that blue cuff thing the doctor had given me. I'd blow the bulb up and sometimes, especially in the beginning, I had to do it over because I failed to gauge the beats correctly or because I hadn't heard a thing. I practiced then on anyone who came. Nobody had ever seen blood pressure as high as yours. You were exceptional, divine, 'a genius' as your sisters said. Poor Zouzou! How we bothered you, telling you all day long to try to eat or drink! You politely refused, but you did refuse. 'No thank you' to everything. I know it was because you couldn't.

"But that's right—for two days you felt like eating peaches. It was a little bit of an extravagance in the month of May. And we were beside ourselves with joy. Yaya brought you some, preciously burrowed into a nest of very soft, very thin straw. I added sugar to make them a little more nourishing, but not so much you would be nauseated, and you nibbled a little—oh, not much. Then you chose a straw, a different color each day, and you drank water in tiny, prudent sips, drops of water. We were on guard a few moments. You didn't move at all, your head pressed to your blue pillow. I'd say, 'Zouzou, tighten your lips, be selfish, keep it for yourself, please, I beg you.' When you suddenly had that look which meant, 'I'm sorry, I can't do otherwise,' and when you clapped your hand to your mouth, I knew that this time again there would be nothing, nothing in your stomach. It refused everything, that heartburn that ceaselessly caused you pain.

"How it all must have bored you, sometimes, even our solicitude. Constant heartburn, vomiting day after day, how painful it must have been, my poor child!

"You weren't very happy when we left for the Le Mans car races, but it was only just for one day. Besides, it was a foolish thing to do; do you remember in what shape, filthy and tired, we got back? And you, you had been much quieter watching the race on TV. And you had a beautiful surprise that day because Françoise Sagan came to see you. Your sisters teased you afterwards, saying, 'What did she say?' and most of all, 'What did you say back? What did you say yourself?' You shrugged your shoulders, 'None of your business!' You are right, Zouk, it was none of their business and, after all, I'm going to tell you a secret, maybe they were jealous.

"You were funny also when your grandmother asked you who had come to see you; you assumed your mysterious little air and answered, 'A writer.'

"I remember that it was the day after your confirmation. It had been very tiring for you, although fortunately you had been excused from part of the ceremony. It was long enough and hot enough as it was. You were very straight and dignified beside your two grandmothers. There was a crowd of little girls and the bishop stopped before each of you, asking your first names, and making a little speech on the corresponding saint.

"I remember that there were so many 'Nathalies' he didn't know what to say any longer, and his delivery somewhat dried up when he came to the twelfth. Saint Anne particularly inspired him, but for the little girl just before you. For you, Zouzou, he had therefore only a few nice words stressing what he had just said, and there was the holy chrism which made a shiny spot on your forehead. Do you know what I felt like saying at that moment? Well, I felt like saying, 'My Lord Bishop, you have just confirmed a saint.' Yes, yes, that's exactly how it was, that's what I felt like saying, because it's true. You smile? You feel like pointing your finger at your temple and making that gesture, turning your hand?

"In fact, when Zoulette returned to see the priest to

whom you both went for confession, he said, 'She had no sins at all.'

"My poor love, you often found us a little crazy. You held nothing against us, of course, but you didn't like some of our silly, sometimes irreverent jokes. Forgive me for having shocked you with all that.

"When you were little, it was easier to cheat, for instance when we didn't go to mass. We'd say, 'We went at six in the morning, or at midnight.' Later, you weren't taken in and you asked no questions.

"Do you remember the day of your first communion? All the little girls were in front, their parents seated in back, the mothers on one side and the fathers on the other. At the time of the communion, after all of you had finished, the mothers around me rose and broke ranks to go to communion. I was the only one not to move. Not that I didn't feel a little silly, planted there all alone. Suddenly, you turned your head and you looked at me. So I too went to communion. You winked at me and gave me a smile when I passed by.

"I still wonder how I could have hesitated a single moment, have risked a single moment to hurt or confuse you, to upset you when the choice was so evident. So simple.

"You were happy, that last weekend in June, when I took you to Orly to take a plane to join Zoulette in Saint-Brieuc.

"You wore your beige suit. It really fitted you, you know. You looked like a little woman and Zoulette found you very elegant when you arrived. That's the day you reached fifteen. Zoulette told me that the flowery telegram pleased you very much and that you helped her make your birthday cake. You must have really enjoyed yourselves, the two of you, cooking in the little house.

"But, that lousy blood pressure which brutally went up over there—230, that's high—so three days later you came back.

"You always had stomachaches, you always had heartburn, but you were becoming slender, pretty, pretty. You remember how Caroline's and Laurence's friends who used to come to the house thought you very pretty. And they told you so. There was even one who promised to take you, you alone, with him to the movies as soon as you felt better, and another who brought you flowers.

"July 9, Uncle René died from terrible abdominal pains, and you said, 'I hope I don't have the same thing he had.' Of course not, you didn't have the same thing he had. You were grieved that day.

"You remember the time I had an awful hangover and I stayed the whole day lying beside you in my large bed, where, by the way, you made yourself at home. You were the one who looked after me all day long; it was really nice of you to fix the cushions under my poor head and bring me glasses of ice water. You possessed me totally that day, didn't you?

"You smile? I know what's in your mind: that it happened other times.

"I adore you, my accomplice.

"You liked to be in my blue room. Sometimes I spread myself out, half on the rug, half on the balcony, or I typed an article my legs folded under me and I got cramps. From time to time you spoke to me and I'd look at you but not answer. I was thinking of something else. Ten minutes later I'd give you an answer. 'Ah? You heard?' you'd say. And nothing more. Your sisters, when something like that happens, *they* always say, 'Pfft! you're not interested? All right, we won't say anything anymore to you.' It's true it's annoying.

"Nanou, it was bad now this fever, and this heart, not the one of the heartburn, the real one, the one we speak of in love, it began to 'gallop.'

"Bombom made you laugh when she came to see you, because she sunbathed almost naked on the balcony. No matter, nobody was there then, either on the side or up there in front. She told you about her maladies, making fun of herself, 'Anne, you understand, I'm a hypochondriac,' she said. You, you smiled.

"In spite of everything, you never missed a thing on TV; you'd gather some strength at the precise moment, duly checked in advance (I'm teasing you), slip out of bed, and by little steps in your bare feet, your cushion under your arm, you went and made yourself comfortable on the yellow sofa to watch the films. You remember: a long time ago we teased you about a series called *Father Knows Best,* and we always called you 'Madame Buckley.'

"Madame Buckley here, Madame Buckley there.

" 'You're a pain in the ass!' you shouted. So we stopped.

"July 14, we had the impression there were only the two of us in Paris. In fact it was almost true. Caroline got back in the evening from the country with a friend who brought you a few big pink roses, the kind that grow any old way, in gardens, or climbing old walls. Later, we squatted on the rug in the big ones' room. Through the window we could make out the Eiffel Tower and, therefore, the fireworks. We stared at that corner of the sky aglow with different colors, but to tell the truth we didn't see much.

"The sixteenth, Zoulette came back for a few days. We didn't know at what time she'd come, but suddenly you said to me, 'She's coming.' We hadn't heard a thing, neither the elevator nor the door. However a few moments later there she was. 'I heard your taxi,' you said when I told her. I had work to do, but I was unable to do it. No sooner had I left the house than I wanted to come back. People found me absent, vague. Everything was indifferent to me and seemed futile aside from you. I was anguished at stealing time from you. Therefore I left people without any explanation and came home quickly, quickly.

"Before leaving again on the twenty-sixth, Zoulette asked that photos be taken of you, because you were so pretty and she wanted to bring some to show her friends in Binic. How right she was! You remember? We spent part of the afternoon bombarding you, Daddy with his Leica and me with your Polaroid. Zoulette took a picture with her; she particularly liked it because the only thing one saw were your big eyes and that very gentle, slightly sad look of yours. *You* weren't pleased because you thought you 'looked sick' in the picture.

"You really made us laugh that evening when, though you hadn't drunk or eaten anything for a long time, you had such beauty and extreme weakness, and you suddenly got impatient because Caroline hadn't heard you call her, or hadn't answered right away, and you thundered with an unheard-of force in your voice, 'Well! Damn it! Are you deaf or what, Caroline? Come and see Mickey Mouse!' You know, we looked at one another then, and we said, 'She's better; she's unbelievable.' Kakoze was there, too. 'She'll be going on all eight again,' she laughed.

"And that other night—a very short time ago—when, as we were having dinner, I heard you hiccup. I stood up and I took the curve of the table at such a speed that I skidded on my clogs and went sprawling on the floor, bumping into everything. Caroline held the basin while you vomited; and I, shaken by a terrible, uncontrollable laughter, I felt for my bumps. Laurence was crying, my falling down had so scared her, and Daddy observed the whole operation. He had a pretty tough time with us, poor man; don't you think so, Zouk?

"You were deep in two books at that time.

"*Je Sais Tout,* that big book Grandma gave you and that entranced you. It was quite heavy, so you propped it up with pillows in order to read it in bed.

"I remember well that the story you liked best was 'The Mystery of the *Marie-Céleste.*' You told me about it. Also the book opens at the right page all by itself.

"The other one was *15 Westerns.* Bombom's last gift. The fringed leather bookmark is at page 143, the chapter called 'Among the Grizzlies and the Osage Indians.'

"You didn't have time to finish it.

"You left.

"And I couldn't keep you from going.

"We couldn't make you wait any longer. A little longer.

"You know, Zouk, I have still a lot of things to tell you, to say to you. But there's no time given us.

"Time??

"But haven't you always known that only love counts?

"You know, Nanou . . . I love you."

La Chèze, August–September, 1971